Retinopathy of Prematurity

Andrés Kychenthal B. · Paola Dorta S.
Editors

Retinopathy of Prematurity

Current Diagnosis and Management

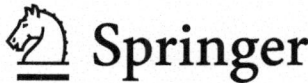 Springer

Editors
Andrés Kychenthal B., MD
KYDOFT
Santiago
Chile

Paola Dorta S., MD, MHA
KYDOFT
Santiago
Chile

ISBN 978-3-319-84843-3   ISBN 978-3-319-52190-9   (eBook)
DOI 10.1007/978-3-319-52190-9

Printed on acid-free paper

This Springer imprint is published by Springer Nature
The registered company is Springer International Publishing AG
The registered company address is: Gewerbestrasse 11, 6330 Cham, Switzerland

Contents

Contributors

Michael P. Blair MD Retina Consultants, LTD, Des Plaines, IL, USA

Antonio Capone, Jr. MD Department of Opthalmology, Associated Retinal Consultants, William Beaumont School of Medicine, Oakland University, Royal Oak, MI, USA

George Caputo MD Department of Pediatric Ophthalmology, Rothschild Ophthalmological Foundation, Paris, France

Paola Dorta S. MD, MHA Ophthalmology, KYDOFT Foundation, Santiago, Chile

Anna L. Ells MD, FRSCS (C) Department of Surgery, University of Calgary, Calgary, AB, Canada

María Eliana Eberhard MD Anesthesia and Pain Unit, Universidad Del Desarollo, Clinica Alemana de Santiago, Santiago, Region Metropolitana, Chile

Alistair R. Fielder FRCP, FRCOphth Optometry & Visual Science, City University London, London, UK

Jose Maria Garcia Gonzalez MD Retina Consultants, LTD, Des Plaines, IL, USA

Mary Elizabeth Hartnett MD Ophthalmology and Visual Sciences, University of Utah/John A. Moran Eye Center, Salt Lake City, UT, USA

Jane Z. Kuo MD, PhD Department of Ophthalmology, Shiley Eye Institute, University of California, San Diego, La Jolla, CA, USA

Andrés Kychenthal B. MD Ophthalmology, KYDOFT Foundation, Santiago, Chile

Thomas Lee MD Ophthalmology Department, The Vision Center, Children's Hospital Los Angeles, Los Angeles, CA, USA

Patricio A. Leyton MD Anestesiología, Clínica Alemana de Santiago, Santiago, Región Metropolitana, Chile

Ramiro S. Maldonado MD Ophthalmology, Duke University, Durham, NC, USA

Monica Morgues Neonatologist Pediatric Department, Campus North, Universidad de Chile/San José Hospital, Santiago, Chile

Anand Muthiah MBBS, MBA, MPH Claremont, CA, USA

Anika Muthiah MBBS Claremont, CA, USA

Eric Nudleman MD, PhD Department of Ophthalmology, Shiley Eye Institute, University of California, San Diego, La Jolla, CA, USA

Adam L. Rothman BS Ophthalmology, Duke University, Durham, NC, USA

Michael J. Shapiro MD Retina Consultants, LTD, Des Plaines, IL, USA

Khaled Tawansy MD Children's Retina Institute, Pasadena, CA, USA

Cynthia A. Toth MD Ophthalmology and Biomedical Engineering, Duke University, Durham, NC, USA

Michael T. Trese MD Eye Research Institute, Oakland University Associated Retinal Consultants, Royal Oak, MI, USA

Lejla Vajzovic MD Ophthalmology, Duke University, Durham, NC, USA

Clare M. Wilson PhD, FRCOphth Ophthalmology, Chelsea and Westminster, London, UK

Wei-Chi Wu MD, PhD Ophthalmology, Chang Gung Memorial Hospital, Kweishan, Taoyuan, Taiwan

Pathophysiology of ROP

Mary Elizabeth Hartnett

Keywords

Preterm · Angiogenesis · Retinopathy of prematurity (ROP) · Vasopro-liferation · Vascular endothelial growth factor (VEGF)

Retinal Vascular Development

It is difficult to study human retinal vascular development because vascularization occurs before term birth, and it is difficult to obtain quality human fetal tissue. Therefore, most studies of retinal vascular development are from newborn animals that vascularize their retinas after term birth. However, there are differences between species, and therefore it is important to review studies that have been done in human eyes [1, 2].

Studies in fetal human tissue provide evidence that the initial vasculature of the retina develops in the posterior pole covering at least the region of zone I through the process of vasculogenesis, or development of vessels from de novo precursors. The precursors migrate from the deep, neuroblastic layers of the retina to the inner surface and become angioblasts. The process begins at about 15-week gestation [2] and continues until at least 22-week gestation, after which insufficient human data are available. After 22-week gestation, it is assumed that the inner and deep retinal vascular plexi develop

through angiogenesis from existing angioblasts or endothelial cells, based on animal models [3, 4]. In addition, Müller cells [5, 6] and other neurons, such as ganglion cells [7] are also important in retinal vascular development.

In human preterm birth, retinal vascular development is incomplete. Additional aspects of premature birth and the stresses surrounding it and the neonatal period, cause abnormal retinal vascular development, manifested first as delayed physiologic retinal vascular development, and later with aberrant vasoproliferation into the vitreous instead of into the retina. These are the refined phases of human ROP (Fig. 1.1) [8].

Term Versus Preterm Birth

To understand what goes wrong in retinopathy of prematurity (ROP), it is helpful to review some of the relevant and known events that occur in normal versus preterm birth, including the roles of oxygen and oxidative stress, and nutritional deficiencies, which have been linked to ROP.

Oxygen

In utero, it has been estimated that oxygen to the developing fetus is about 30–40 mm Hg, so the ambient environment after birth is relatively hyperoxic, particularly when supplemental

M.E. Hartnett (✉)
Ophthalmology and Visual Sciences, University of Utah/John A. Moran Eye Center, 65 Mario Capecchi Dr, Salt Lake City, UT 84132, USA
e-mail: me.hartnett@hsc.utah.edu

© Springer International Publishing AG 2017
Andrés Kychenthal B. and Paola Dorta S. (eds.), *Retinopathy of Prematurity*,
DOI 10.1007/978-3-319-52190-9_1

Fig. 1.1 Phases of human
ROP. Drawing by James
Gilman, CRA, FOPS. From
ophthalmology, 2015
Jan;122(1):200–10,
Hartnett ME,
pathophysiology and
mechanisms of severe
retinopathy of prematurity

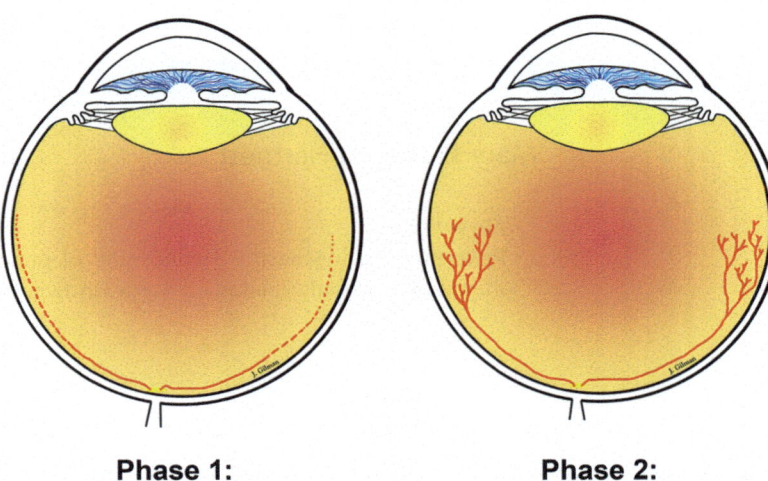

Phase 1:
Delayed Physiological
Retinal Vascular Development

Phase 2:
Vaso-proliferation

oxygen is used for resuscitation [9]. High oxygen at birth has been shown to cause vasoattenuation and death to newly formed endothelial cells, [10] creating areas of retina devoid of capillary support. Human preterm infants in the US exposed to 100% oxygen prior to the technologic advances for monitoring and regulating oxygen, developed retrolental fibroplasia (RLF), now believed to be stage 5, the worst form of ROP [11]. The appearance of a white pupil represented a retrolental fibrovascular scar with an underlying retinal detachment. What actually occurred in the preterm infant retina prior to the development of RLF was limited because the Schepens/Pomerantzeff binocular indirect ophthalmoscope and other methods to observe the peripheral retina had not been widely adopted [12]. Therefore, experimental approaches using newborn animals exposed to conditions similar to what preterm infants then experienced were analyzed. From early experiments, it was hypothesized that high oxygen-induced capillary loss and avascular retina, and that removal from supplemental oxygen to ambient air, caused the avascular retina to become hypoxic and release angiogenic factors that led to aberrant angiogenesis and scarring [10]. These experiments also led to a phased approach description of ROP: phase 1, representing vasoobliteration, phase 2, vasoproliferation and phase 3, a fibrovascular phase in

human and not animal models associated with retinal detachment [13]. When oxygen level was reduced, RLF virtually disappeared [11], but at too low an oxygen level there was increased risk of cerebral palsy and death [14]. Now, countries that lack resources for prenatal and perioperative care and oxygen regulation report ROP and hyperoxia-induced vasoattenuation, documented by fluorescein angiography, in large and older gestational aged infants than those in the US [15]. Advancements in neonatal care and oxygen regulation and monitoring have permitted infants of lower birth weights and younger gestational ages to survive. In countries implementing these changes, ROP is seen in infants of extremely low birth weight (<1000 g) and gestational ages (<28 wks), and the two-phase description of ROP has been refined to be delayed physiologic retinal vascular development with some vasoattenuation in phase 1 and vasoproliferation in phase 2.

Oxygen Stresses and Oxidation

The mechanisms whereby high oxygen affects newly developed capillaries and endothelial cells are not completely understood. Although the sensitivity of endothelial cells for oxygen lessens with development, hyperoxia-induced endothelial cell damage has still been reported in adult mice [16]. One potential mechanism whereby high oxygen damages endothelial cells is from mitochondrial-generated reactive oxygen species (ROS). In addition, other oxygen stresses, including fluctuations in oxygenation [17] and intermittent hypoxia [18], may lead to ROS generated from other sources, such as the activation of NADPH oxidase, a leading generator of ROS in endothelial cells. Also, reactive nitrogen species from activation of endothelial nitric oxide synthetase (eNOS) can generate nitric oxide (NO), which under certain circumstances forms damaging reactive nitrogen species (RNS), including peroxynitrite [19]. Nitric oxide can be beneficial to the preterm lungs and as an endothelial relaxing agent, and ROS are important in metabolism and for fighting invading microorganisms, but too many ROS or RNS can also cause direct tissue damage or indirect pathology from abnormal activation of signaling pathways. Generally, the reactive compounds are kept in check through antioxidant enzymes or nonenzymatic mechanisms, but the loss of balance between antioxidants and reactive species can lead to damage. There is evidence suggesting an imbalance occurs in preterm infants. Compared to infants born full-term, premature infants consume more glutathione (GSH), which provides a nonenzymatic oxidative reserve in red blood cells [20]. Hypoxia in complicated births is also believed to reduce the ability to quench mitochondrial ROS trapping [21]. In studies done in neonatal piglets, there is evidence that prostaglandins, such as E2, help preserve neural function following episodes of hypoxia, what occurs during progressive labor, but this mechanism may not be sufficient in abrupt preterm birth [22]. Also, preterm infants may be unable to express antioxidant enzymes until later age.

In regions that regulate oxygen, fluctuations in oxygenation have been measured in preterm infants in association with increased risk of ROP [17]. Fluctuations between 50 and 10% inspired oxygen in newborn rats cause similar arterial oxygen extremes in preterm infants and delayed physiologic retinal vascular development in experimental models, in part through the generation of ROS from activated NADPH oxidase [23–25] that causes endothelial cell death. Activation of NADPH oxidase in endothelial cells can also lead to vasoproliferation in a similar model of oxygen fluctuations [26].

Oxygen Trials

The practicality of regulating oxygen as a treatment for ROP has been tested in several multicenter clinical trials, including the Supplemental Therapeutic Oxygen to Prevent ROP (STOP-ROP) study [27], Surfactant Positive Airway Pressure Pulse Oximetry Randomized Trial (SUPPORT), Benefits of Oxygen Saturation Targeting Study II (BOOST II), and Canadian Oxygen Trial (COT) [28]. STOP-ROP failed to find a significant reduction in ROP from oxygen saturations between 96 and 99% when delivered for prethreshold ROP compared to 89–94%, except in a subgroup without evidence of plus disease [27]. Other clinical studies have reported either increased [29, 30] or decreased risk [31, 32] of ROP from high oxygen. The SUPPORT and BOOST II randomized clinical trials reported that oxygen saturation targets between 85 and 89% compared to 91–95% saturation were associated with increased mortality, but survivors of 85–89% oxygen saturation had a lower incidence of ROP. In the COT, which tested similar oxygen saturation targets in preterm infants of the same gestational ages, as did SUPPORT and BOOSTII, there was no difference in ROP or mortality. The COT was performed later in time from infants in different regions of the world compared to SUPPORT or BOOSTII, and also excluded from enrollment infants with pulmonary hypertension. From these studies, there does not appear to be consensus as to appropriate and safe oxygen saturation targets for preterm infants. The practicality of safely regulating oxygen in the individual preterm infant can be difficult because phases of ROP are not as distinct as in experimental models, and oxygen affects other organs in the developing preterm infant [28], and ongoing analyses from these studies are underway.

Nutrition

Much of the nutritional support to the fetus occurs in the last trimester, such that when an infant is born prematurely, maternal support is lost [33]. Studies have shown the importance of insulin-like growth factor (IGF-1) and insulin-like growth factor binding protein 3 (IGF-1BP3) [34, 35] to infant development, which are reduced in the preterm infant in association with delayed physiologic retinal vascular development. In addition, omega-3 fatty acids, which make up the phospholipid rich tissue in neurons in the brain and photoreceptors in the retina, are reduced. Studies are ongoing to determine if recombinant human IGF-1 and IGF-1BP3 (rhIGF-I/rhIGFBP-3) will reduce ROP in infants. The phases in human ROP are not as distinct as in experimental models and there is concern that rhIGF-I/rhIGFBP-3 may be given to an infant who is about to develop vasoproliferative phase but who does not manifest signs of it. To reduce this, attempts are in place to increase the IGF-1/IGF-1BP3 only to levels normally found in infants of the gestational ages. Omega-3 FAs, if effective, can reduce both phase 1 and 2 in experimental models [36].

Phases of ROP and Phases of Experimental Oxygen-Induced Retinopathy

The initial two-phase hypothesis of human ROP described in the 1950s was based in large part on animal models in which retinal vascularization occurred after birth. Nonetheless, it is impossible to experiment on human preterm infant eyes safely and study mechanisms of human ROP; therefore, models of oxygen-induced retinopathy (OIR) are essential. It is important to consider the experimental question carefully when choosing a model or models (Fig. 1.2). The most representative model of human ROP today is the rat OIR model [37], which varies oxygen exposure between 50 and 10% to newborn rat pups and has been recently adapted to study molecular mechanisms using gene therapy techniques [6, 38–40]. Most studies have used the mouse OIR model, which exposes day 7 animals with inner plexus vascularization to high oxygen in order to damage already developed capillaries [41]. The mouse model is robust to study mechanisms of high oxygen-induced stress through the use of transgenic animals. The beagle OIR model uses high oxygen but is more similar to human ROP in that the retina continues to develop after birth. The beagle OIR model is also useful to translate pharmacologic interventions since the puppy eye size is closer to the human infant than is a rodent eye [42, 43].

Role of VEGF and Angiogenesis

Physiologic hypoxia is important in upregulating VEGF locally to promote normal retinal vascular development [4, 44, 45]. The parent VEGF mRNA has splice variants that have different biologic properties believed partly related to whether the translated proteins are cell associated, soluble, or have both characteristics [46]. VEGF splice variants are important in development and in aberrant angiogenesis. VEGF165 is both cell associated and can affect other retinal cells through soluble properties. VEGF164 (the analog of human VEGF165) is involved in vascular development in mice [47], but is upregulated by repeated fluctuations in oxygenation similar to the extremes in arterial oxygen in preterm infants who develop severe ROP [17]. In contrast, hypoxia alone increases the expression of soluble VEGF120 [25]. Inhibition of the rat VEGF164 [48] with a neutralizing antibody or by targeted gene therapy to introduce a shRNA to knock down VEGF164 only in Müller cells, reduced vasoproliferation but not physiologic retinal vascular development in the rat OIR model [6].

VEGF binds its receptors and triggers signaling of biochemical cascades to cause biologic events. There are three receptors and VEGFR2 is believed to be involved in much of the pathologic angiogenesis, although VEGFR1 is also important. Some studies support the idea that regulation of

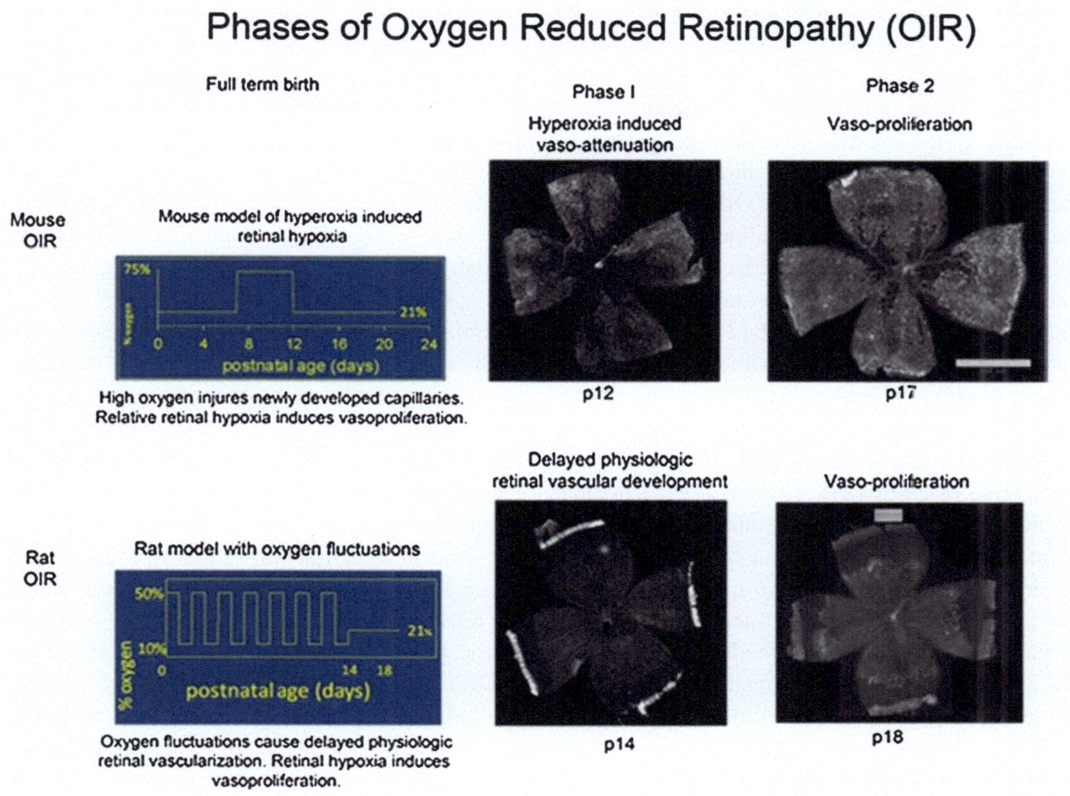

Phases of Oxygen Reduced Retinopathy (OIR)

Full term birth

Mouse OIR

Mouse model of hyperoxia induced retinal hypoxia

High oxygen injures newly developed capillaries. Relative retinal hypoxia induces vasoproliferation.

Phase I
Hyperoxia induced vaso-attenuation
p12

Phase 2
Vaso-proliferation
p17

Rat OIR

Rat model with oxygen fluctuations

Oxygen fluctuations cause delayed physiologic retinal vascularization. Retinal hypoxia induces vasoproliferation.

Delayed physiologic retinal vascular development
p14

Vaso-proliferation
p18

Fig. 1.2 Phases of oxygen-induced Retinopathy (OIR). From ophthalmology, 2015 Jan;122(1):200–10, Hartnett ME, Pathophysiology and mechanisms of severe retinopathy of prematurity

VEGFR2 signaling is important in ordering developmental angiogenesis. Over activation of VEGFR2 disordered the cleavage planes of dividing vascular cells causing them to take on a disordered pattern of growth [49]. Order was restored in experimental models with a neutralizing antibody to VEGF164 or through gene therapy to knock down Müller cell VEGF164. The evidence supports the notion that disordered endothelial cell growth enables cells to grow outside the plane of the retina and into the vitreous, whereas restoration of physiologic, ordered growth enables intraretinal blood vessel growth and reduces peripheral avascular retina. Over activation of VEGFR2 can occur by interactions with different receptors, such as the erythropoietin receptor (EPOR), or with other proteins including NOX4 [23], an isoform of NADPH oxidase, most likely through adaptor proteins. Downstream activation of the transcription factor, signal transducer, and activator of transcription 3 (STAT3) in endothelial cells causes vasoproliferation in experimental models [26].

Role of Anemia and Erythropoietin

Many preterm infants develop anemia of prematurity related to blood draws, inadequate erythropoiesis, and possible loss of blood at the time of delivery. Studies that tested the effect of restrictive versus liberal blood transfusions found no differences in the development of ROP [50, 51].

Erythropoietin (EPO) and its derivatives, such as darbepoietin, have been used for anemia of prematurity, but some clinical studies have associated severe ROP with the use of EPO [19, 20].

Vitreous EPO was increased in infants who underwent vitrectomies for stage 4 ROP compared to cataract surgery [21]. However, a recent clinical trial in infants given darbepoietin for neuroprotection found no effect compared to control on severe ROP [52], although, the number of infants with severe ROP was small. In addition, experimental studies found EPO administered early can stabilize newly formed retinal capillaries [23] and encourage physiologic retinal vascular development [24], but if given late can contribute to vasoproliferation [17, 22]. There is renewed interest in EPO for neuroprotection. EPO receptor can dimerize with itself or with the beta common receptor to form a tissue protective receptor [28]. However, experimental studies in the rat OIR model found very little beta common receptor expression in the retina in room air raised pups or those in the OIR model [40]. In contrast, repeated fluctuations in oxygenation activated not only the EPO receptor but also VEGFR2, which together formed a heterodimer and caused vitreous vasoproliferation in phase 2. Also, EPO was not increased in the OIR model but both EPOR expression and activation were increased. Furthermore, not only did EPO activate its receptor but VEGF also activated EPOR. With increasing expression of VEGF by oxygen stresses in ROP or through exogenous delivery of EPO, EPOR may be activated and interact with VEGFR2 to increase vasoproliferation. These observations may partly explain the discrepancies reported on EPO use in ROP. As with IGF-1 and other angiogenic factors that can reduce phase 1 ROP, the timing of delivery of the angiogenic agent, to avoid vasoproliferation, is complicated in the individual infant in whom the phases of ROP are not distinct.

Role of Oxidation, Inflammation, and Angiogenesis

Oxygen levels affect oxidation and the generation of ROS and RNS through mitochondria, NADPH oxidase, eNOS, and other enzymes. In addition, oxidative reserve is less in preterm than in full-term infants. High oxygen can increase the superoxide radical, and low oxygen may also increase superoxide [53] by slowing upstream events in the electron transport chain and increasing the concentration of oxygen donors. Repeated oxygen fluctuations can also activate enzymes that generate ROS, including NADPH oxidase. In addition, infection and inflammation can lead to signaling events that overlap with oxidative signaling [54], including angiogenesis and apoptosis [55, 56].

Inflammatory compounds are increased in low birth weight preterm infants in the antenatal period [57]. One family of metabolites includes the phospholipase A2 (PLA-2) enzymes that catalyze the hydrolysis of fatty acids from membrane phospholipids and are activated by oxidative stresses and hypoxia. PLA-2 is involved in experimental retinal neovascularization [58]. Activation of PLA-2 can then lead to the release of arachidonic acid, platelet activating factor, and lysophospholipids. Cyclo oxygenases (COX1 and COX2) can oxidize and catalyze arachidonic acid into the eicosanoids, including prostaglandins, prostacyclin, and thromboxanes that have been associated with both avascular retina and vasoproliferation in models of ROP and OIR [58]. Prostaglandin E2 activation of its receptor, EP4, caused Müller cell overexpression of VEGF and vasoproliferation in experimental OIR models [59].

Hypoxia, ROS, and inflammatory pathways through NFkB can stabilize hypoxia-inducible factor alpha 1 alpha (HIF1α). HIF1α then translocates to the nucleus initiating transcription of a number of angiogenic genes, including VEGF, erythropoietin, and angiopoietin 2, as examples [60]. HIF1α can also upregulate RTP801 to induce angiogenesis in a pathway independent of VEGF. RTP801 is strongly upregulated in ischemic cells of neuronal origin and can cause neuronal apoptosis [61]. Hypoxia also can increase the Krebs cycle metabolite, succinate, in retinal ganglion cells and trigger signaling through its receptor, GRPR91, to affect developmental angiogenesis and vasoproliferation in OIR models [7].

The cytochrome p450 monooxygenases (CYP) include a number of oxygen sensitive proteins that oxidize compounds, notably arachidonic acid. Autooxidation of arachidonic acid via CYP can produce lipid peroxides. CYP1B1 was also found to increase anti-angiogenic agent, thrombospondin 2 [62]. There is some evidence that CYP activation can exacerbate phospholipase A2 dependent injury [63] and may lead to a pathway associated with hyperoxia-induced endothelial apoptosis and vasoobliteration, seen in the mouse OIR model [64]. These events can contribute to avascular retina.

Generation of RNS, including peroxynitrite, can damage tissue but its precursor, NO, can be beneficial, and the difference may be related to the redox state of the tissue [65]. Other RNS, such as NO_2^*, can lead to the isomerization of arachidonic acid to trans-arachidonic acid. Trans-arachidonic acid has been shown to contribute to hyperoxia-induced vasoobliteration through the upregulation of anti-angiogenic agent, thrombospondin-1 [56].

Although experimental approaches have shown that antioxidants can improve physiologic retinal vascular development, they have not reduced vasoproliferation. In human infants, antioxidants, n-acetyl cysteine [66], vitamin E [67] or lutein [68] also failed to safely reduce severe ROP. There can be different effects of ROS in different cells and evidence suggests that this is why broad inhibition of ROS may not always yield expected outcomes. In a rat OIR model in which rats were placed into 28% supplemental oxygen (supplemental oxygen OIR model) instead of room air, the antioxidant, apocynin, reduced vasoproliferation in part by inhibiting STAT3. In addition, vasoproliferation was nearly abolished with a systemic or intravitreal STAT3 inhibitor. However, in the rat OIR model in which rats were placed into room air (standard OIR model), broad STAT3 inhibition had no effect on vasoproliferation. The reason appeared to be based on the cell type in which STAT3 was activated. In contrast to the events in the supplemental oxygen OIR model, activation of STAT3 occurred in Müller cells by high VEGF in the standard OIR model and led to downregulation of EPO and delayed physiologic retinal vascular development. Exogenous EPO

increased physiologic retinal vascular development by 40% but did not reduce vasoproliferation in phase 2, possibly because of the angiogenic effects of EPO. In the supplemental oxygen OIR model, VEGF was relatively downregulated compared to the standard OIR model reducing the effect of Müller cell STAT3 on EPO downregulation. In the supplemental oxygen OIR model, NADPH oxidase induced STAT3 was activated in endothelial cells and inhibition of STAT3 reduced vasoproliferation [26]. In the standard OIR model, STAT3 activation by VEGF mediated VEGFR2 activation in endothelial cells was in part through NADPH oxidase [26], as seen with high glucose [69]. This evidence supports the notion that reduction in vasoproliferation requires targeted endothelial cell STAT3 inhibition because broad inhibition of STAT3 may lead to upregulation of EPO that can act as an angiogenic factor. Studies are ongoing to look at ways to increase the effect of hypoxia inducible factors to support physiologic vascularization of the retina during high oxygen when hypoxia inducible factors are turned off during high oxygen treatment, which is often necessary for survival of the premature infant [70]. However, greater study is needed because many of these factors also affect processes important to the premature infant.

VEGF Signaling

Over activation of VEGF in the retina can disorder developmental angiogenesis and cause not only vasoproliferation into the vitreous, but also delayed physiologic retinal vascular development in phase 1. Inhibition of VEGF signaling can facilitate physiologic vascular development while inhibiting vasoproliferation. This finding was also seen in the clinical trial, Bevacizumab Eliminates the Angiogenic Threat of ROP (BEAT-ROP). However, in some infants treated with bevacizumab, persistent avascular retina and later vasoproliferation occurred. Concerns exist that the dose of anti-VEGF agent, which was based on adult sized eyes, was too great for the preterm infant eye. In addition, the dilution of anti-VEGF agent that enters the blood volume in the preterm infant is much less than in the adult, and VEGF is important in neuroprotection, lung, and kidney development. More studies are needed to determine dose and safety.

Experimental data from OIR models also show adverse effects even with Müller cell targeted knockdown of VEGF at a dose to significantly inhibit vasoproliferation, but not physiologic retinal vascular development. As an example, targeted inhibition of VEGFA in Müller cells with lentivector gene therapy reduced the capillary density of the inner and deep plexi of the retina even though the extent of vascular coverage was not affected [39]. This treatment also caused neural death and later thinning of the outer nuclear layer. Neutralizing VEGF164 with an antibody led to recurrent vasoproliferation at a later time point in the rat OIR model in association with upregulation of other angiogenic pathways and with inhibition of pup body weight gain [71]. Both interventions, targeting VEGF in Müller cells only with the lentivector gene therapy or using an antibody to VEGF164, reduced vasoproliferation in the rat OIR model fourfold compared to each respective control, but both anti-VEGF strategies led to adverse events in the developing retina and rat pup. These findings raise the question whether inhibition of the growth factor VEGF may be too extreme a treatment for the developing preterm infant and eye. Experimental studies that introduced a short hairpin RNA to knock down VEGF164 in Müller cells only showed efficacy at inhibiting vasoproliferation without causing cell death or thinning of the ONL [6].

Additional considerations regarding anti-VEGF agents are important. The phenotype of ROP varies throughout the world based on resources for care and oxygen delivery. Infants in India who develop severe ROP are born at older gestational ages (>32 weeks) and larger birth weights than infants even screened in countries with resources for oxygen regulation and care. These larger and older preterm infants differ substantially from preterm infants who develop severe ROP in the US. Therefore, studies of anti-VEGF agents may not be comparable between the US and areas in which older and larger preterm infants are treated with anti-VEGF agents.

The Role of Light

The Light-ROP study tested the hypothesis that light would generate harmful ROS and cause ROP in newly born infants. However, there was no effect on the development of prethreshold ROP in infants that wore goggles to reduce light to the retinas [72]. A study found that mice reared in the dark in utero developed characteristics that may predispose the retina to the development of ROP [73]. Light induced the maturation of a particular type of ganglion cells, the melanopsin ganglion cells. Evidence was presented in human preterm infants that higher average day length during early gestation was associated with lower risk of ROP [74]. Finally, a large candidate study of extremely low birth weight infants found two variants in the gene encoding brain-derived neurotrophic factor (BDNF) were associated with severe ROP. Additional studies are needed to understand the links between light level and physiologic retinal vascular development.

Summary

ROP differs throughout the world and is affected by a number of factors: prenatal care, nutritional support, oxygenation levels, inflammation, infection, and oxidation. VEGF is an important factor in developmental and pathologic angiogenesis. Oxidative signaling is also important but leads to different outcomes in different cells. Use of angiogenic agonists to promote physiologic retinal vascular development may be of concern in the preterm infant, in whom the phases of ROP are not distinct. However, angiogenic inhibitors are also of concern since the determination of dose will be challenging and cannot be compared between studies of large and small preterm infants. Recent evidence suggests that regulating VEGF receptor signaling at the endothelial cell or inhibiting signaling effectors downstream of VEGFR2 using targeted approaches may be important.

References

1. Chan-Ling T, McLeod DS, Hughes S, Baxter L, Chu Y, Hasegawa T, et al. Astrocyte-endothelial cell relationships during human retinal vascular development. Invest Ophthalmol Vis Sci. 2004;45(6):2020–32.
2. McLeod DS, Hasegawa T, Prow T, Merges C, Lutty G. The initial fetal human retinal vasculature develops by vasculogenesis. Dev Dyn. 2006;235 (12):3336–47. doi:10.1002/dvdy.20988.
3. Dorrell MI, Aguilar E, Friedlander M. Retinal vascular development is mediated by endothelial filopodia, a preexisting astrocytic template and specific R-cadherin adhesion. Invest Ophthalmol Vis Sci. 2002;43(11):3500–10.
4. Chan-Ling T, Gock B, Stone J. The effect of oxygen on vasoformative cell division: evidence that 'physiological hypoxia' is the stimulus for normal retinal vasculogenesis. Invest Ophthalmol Vis Sci. 1995;36:1201–14.
5. Bai Y, J-X Ma, Guo J, Wang J, Zhu M, Chen Y, et al. Müller cell-derived VEGF is a significant contributor to retinal neovascularization. J Pathol. 2009;219(4):446–54.
6. Jiang Y, Wang H, Culp D, Yang Z, Fotheringham L, Flannery J, et al. Targeting Muller cell-derived VEGF164 to reduce intravitreal neovascularization in the rat model of retinopathy of prematurity. Invest Ophthalmol Vis Sci. 2014;55(2):824–31. doi:10. 1167/iovs.13-13755.
7. Sapieha P, Sirinyan M, Hamel D, Zaniolo K, Joyal JS, Cho JH, et al. The succinate receptor GPR91 in neurons has a major role in retinal angiogenesis. Nat Med. 2008;14(10):1067–76.
8. Hartnett ME, Penn JS. Mechanisms and management of retinopathy of prematurity. N Engl J Med. 2012;367(26):2515–26.
9. Saugstad OD, Ramji S, Soll RF, Vento M. Resuscitation of newborn infants with 21% or 100% oxygen: an updated systematic review and meta-analysis. Neonatology. 2008;94(3):176–82. doi:10.1159/0001 43397.
10. Ashton N, Ward B, Serpell G. Effect of oxygen on developing retinal vessels with particular reference to the problem of retrolental fibroplasia. Br J Ophthalmol. 1954;38:397–430.
11. Patz A, Hoeck LE, De La Cruz E. Studies on the effect of high oxygen administration in retrolental fibroplasia. I. Nursery observations. Am J Ophthalmol. 1952;35(9):1248–53.
12. Schepens CL. A new ophthalmoscope demonstration. Trans Am Acad Ophthalmol Otolaryngol. 1947;51:298–301.
13. Hartnett ME. Ophthalmology. 2015 Jan;122(1): 200-10.
14. Patz A. Studies on retinal neovascularization. Friedenwald lecture. Invest Ophthalmol Vis Sci. 1980;19(10):1133–8.
15. Shah PK, Narendran V, Kalpana N. Aggressive posterior retinopathy of prematurity in large preterm babies in South India. Arch Dis Child Fetal Neonatal Ed. 2012;97(5):F371–5. doi:10.1136/fetalneonatal-2011-301121.
16. Yamada H, Yamada E, Hackett SF, Ozaki H, Okamoto N, Campochiaro PA. Hyperoxia causes decreased expression of vascular endothelial growth factor and endothelial cell apoptosis in adult retina. J Cell Physiol. 1999;179(2):149–56. doi:10.1002/ (sici)1097-4652(199905)179:2<149:aid-jcp5>3.0.co;2-2.
17. Cunningham S, Fleck BW, Elton RA, McIntosh N. Transcutaneous oxygen levels in retinopathy of prematurity. Lancet. 1995;346:1464–5.
18. Di Fiore JM, Kaffashi F, Loparo K, Sattar A, Schluchter M, Foglyano R, et al. The relationship between patterns of intermittent hypoxia and retinopathy of prematurity in preterm infants. Pediatr Res. 2012;72(6):606–12. doi:10.1038/pr.2012.132.
19. Brooks SE, Gu X, Samuel S, Marcus DM, Bartoli M, Huang PL, et al. Reduced severity of oxygen-induced retinopathy in eNOS-deficient mice. Invest Ophthalmol Vis Sci. 2001;42:222–8.
20. Buhimschi IA, Buhimschi CS, Pupkin M, Weiner CP. Beneficial impact of term labor: Nonenzymatic antioxidant reserve in the human fetus. Am J Obstet Gynecol. 2003;189(1):181–8.
21. Sanchez-Alvarez ROSA, Almeida A, Medina JM. Oxidative stress in preterm rat brain is due to mitochondrial dysfunction. Pediatr Res. 2002;51(1): 34–9.
22. Najarian T, Hardy P, Hou X, Lachapelle J, Doke A, Gobeil F Jr, et al. Preservation of neural function in the perinate by high PGE2 levels acting via EP2 receptors. J Appl Physiol. 2000;89(2):777–84.
23. Wang H, Yang Z, Jiang Y, Hartnett ME. Endothelial NADPH oxidase 4 mediates vascular endothelial growth factor receptor 2-induced intravitreal neovascularization in a rat model of retinopathy of prematurity. Mol Vis. 2014;20:231–41.
24. Niesman MR, Johnson KA, Penn JS. Therapeutic effect of liposomal superoxide dismutase in an animal model of retinopathy of prematurity. Neurochem Res. 1997;22(5):597–605.
25. McColm JR, Geisen P, Hartnett ME. VEGF isoforms and their expression after a single episode of hypoxia or repeated fluctuations between hyperoxia and hypoxia: relevance to clinical ROP. Mol Vision. 2004;10:512–20.
26. Byfield G, Budd S, Hartnett ME. The role of supplemental oxygen and JAK/STAT signaling in intravitreous neovascularization in a ROP rat model. Invest Ophthalmol Vis Sci. 2009;50(7):3360–5. doi:10.1167/iovs.08-3256.

27. Group TS-RMS. Supplemental therapeutic oxygen for prethreshold retinopathy of prematurity (STOP-ROP), a randomized, controlled trial. I: primary outcomes. Pediatrics. 2000;105(2):295–310.

28. Hartnett ME, Lane RH. Effects of oxygen on the development and severity of retinopathy of prematurity. J AAPOS Official Publ Am Assoc Pediatr Ophthalmol Strabismus/Am Assoc Pediatr Ophthalmol Strabismus. 2013;17(3):229–34. doi:10.1016/j.jaapos.2012.12.155.

29. Vanderveen DK, Mansfield TA, Eichenwald EC. Lower oxygen saturation alarm limits decrease the severity of retinopathy of prematurity. J Am Assoc Pediatr Ophthalmol Strabismus. 2006;10(5):445–8.

30. Wallace DK, Veness-Meehan KA, Miller WC. Incidence of severe retinopathy of prematurity before and after a modest reduction in target oxygen saturation levels. J Am Assoc Pediatr Ophthalmol Strabismus. 2007;11(2):170–4.

31. Sears JE, Pietz J, Sonnie C, Dolcini D, Hoppe G. A change in oxygen supplementation can decrease the incidence of retinopathy of prematurity. Ophthalmology. 2009;116(3):513–8.

32. Gaynon MW. Rethinking stop-rop: is it worthwhile trying to modulate excessive VEGF levels in prethreshold rop eyes by systemic intervention?: A review of the role of oxygen, light adaptation state, and anemia in prethreshold ROP. Retina. 2006;26(7).

33. Hellström A, Smith LEH, Dammann O. Retinopathy of prematurity. Lancet. 2013;382(9902):1445–57.

34. Lofqvist C, Chen J, Connor KM, Smith ACH, Aderman CM, Liu N, et al. From the cover: IGFBP3 suppresses retinopathy through suppression of oxygen-induced vessel loss and promotion of vascular regrowth. Proc Natl Acad Sci. 2007;104(25):10589–94.

35. Chang KH, Chan-Ling T, McFarland EL, Afzal A, Pan H, Baxter LC, et al. IGF binding protein-3 regulates hematopoietic stem cell and endothelial precursor cell function during vascular development. Proc Natl Acad Sci. 2007;104(25):10595–600.

36. Connor KM, SanGiovanni JP, Lofqvist C, Aderman CM, Chen J, Higuchi A, et al. Increased dietary intake of [omega]-3-polyunsaturated fatty acids reduces pathological retinal angiogenesis. Nat Med. 2007;13(7):868–73.

37. Tolman BL, Henry MM, Lowery LA, Penn JS. Oxygen-induced retinopathy in the rat: the period of variable oxygen cycles effects the severity of the pathology. Invest Ophthalmol Vis Sci. 1993;34 (Suppl):838.

38. Wang H, Smith GW, Yang Z, Jiang Y, McCloskey M, Greenberg K, et al. Short hairpin RNA-mediated knockdown of VEGFA in Muller cells reduces intravitreal neovascularization in a rat model of retinopathy of prematurity. Am J Pathol. 2013;. doi:10.1016/j.ajpath.2013.05.011.

39. Wang H, Yang Z, Jiang Y, Flannery J, Hammond S, Kafri T, et al. Quantitative analyses of retinal vascular area and density after different methods to reduce VEGF in a rat model of retinopathy of prematurity. Invest Ophthalmol Vis Sci. 2014;55 (2):737–44. doi:10.1167/iovs.13-13429.

40. Yang Z, Wang H, Jiang Y, Hartnett ME. VEGFA activates erythropoietin receptor and enhances VEGFR2-mediated pathological angiogenesis. Am J Pathol. 2014;184(4):1230–9. doi:10.1016/j.ajpath.2013.12.023.

41. Smith LEH, Wesolowski E, McLellan A, Kostyk SK, D'Amato R, Sullivan R, et al. Oxygen induced retinopathy in the mouse. Invest Ophthalmol Vis Sci. 1994;35(1):101–11.

42. McLeod DS, Crone SN, Lutty GA. Vasoproliferation in the neonatal dog model of oxygen-induced retinopathy. Invest Ophthalmol Vis Sci. 1996;37 (7):1322–33.

43. Lutty GA, McLeod DS, Bhutto I, Wiegand SJ. Effect of VEGF trap on normal retinal vascular development and oxygen-induced retinopathy in the dog. Invest Ophthalmol Vis Sci. 2011;52(7):4039–47.

44. Gerhardt H, Golding M, Fruttiger M, Ruhrberg C, Lundkvist A, Abramsson A, et al. VEGF guides angiogenic sprouting utilizing endothelial tip cell filopodia. J Cell Biol. 2003;161(6):1163–77.

45. Stone J, Itin A, Alon T, Peer J, Gnessin H, Chan-Ling T, et al. Development of retinal vasculature is mediated by hypoxia-induced vascular endothelial growth factor (VEGF) expression by neuroglia. J Neurosci. 1995;15:4738–47.

46. Stalmans I, Ng YS, Rohan R, Fruttiger M, Bouche A, Yuce A, et al. Arteriolar and venular patterning in retinas of mice selectively expressing VEGF isoforms. J Clin Invest. 2002;109(3):327–36.

47. Lundkvist A, Lee S, Iruela-Arispe L, Betsholtz C, Gerhardt H. Growth factor gradients in vascular patterning. Novartis Found Symp. 2007;283:194–201; discussion-6, 38–41.

48. Geisen P, Peterson L, Martiniuk D, Uppal A, Saito Y, Hartnett M. Neutralizing antibody to VEGF reduces intravitreous neovascularization and does not interfere with vascularization of avascular retina in an ROP model. Mol Vision. 2008;14:345–57.

49. Zeng G, Taylor SM, McColm JR, Kappas NC, Kearney JB, Williams LH, et al. Orientation of endothelial cell division is regulated by VEGF signaling during blood vessel formation. Blood. 2007;109(4):1345–52.

50. Bell EF, Strauss RG, Widness JA, Mahoney LT, Mock DM, Seward VJ, et al. Randomized trial of liberal versus restrictive guidelines for red blood cell transfusion in preterm infants. Pediatrics. 2005;115 (6):1685–91.

51. Kirpalani H, Whyte RK, Andersen C, Asztalos EV, Heddle N, Blajchman MA et al. The premature infants in need of transfusion (pint) study: a randomized, controlled trial of a restrictive (LOW) versus liberal (HIGH) transfusion threshold for extremely low birth weight infants. J Pediatr. 2006;149(3):301–7.

52. Ohls RK, Christensen RD, Kamath-Rayne BD, Rosenberg A, Wiedmeier SE, Roohi M, et al. A randomized, masked, placebo-controlled study of darbepoetin Alfa in preterm infants. Pediatrics. 2013. doi:10.1542/peds.2013-0143.

53. Ward JPT. Oxygen sensors in context. Biochimica et Biophysica Acta (BBA)—Bioenergetics. 2008;1777 (1):1–14.

54. Wang H, Zhang SX, Hartnett ME. Signaling pathways triggered by oxidative stress that mediate features of severe retinopathy of prematurity. JAMA Ophthalmol. 2013;131(1):80–5. doi:10.1001/jamaophthalmol.2013.986.

55. Saugstad OD. Oxidative stress in the newborn—a 30-year perspective. Biol Neonate. 2005;88(3):228–36.

56. Kermorvant-Duchemin E, Sapieha P, Sirinyan M, Beauchamp M, Checchin D, Hardy P, et al. Understanding ischemic retinopathies: emerging concepts from oxygen-induced retinopathy. Doc Ophthalmol. 2010;120(1):51–60.

57. Dammann O, Phillips TM, Allred EN, O'Shea TM, Paneth N, Van Marter LJ, et al. Mediators of fetal inflammation in extremely low gestational age newborns. Cytokine. 2001;13(4):234–9.

58. Barnett JM, McCollum GW, Penn JS. Role of cytosolic phospholipase A2 in retinal neovascularization. Invest Ophthalmol Vis Sci. 2010;51(2):1136–42.

59. Yanni SE, Barnett JM, Clark ML, Penn JS. The role of PGE2 receptor EP4 in pathologic ocular angiogenesis. Invest Ophthalmol Vis Sci. 2009;50(11): 5479–86.

60. Rey S, Semenza GL. Hypoxia-inducible factor-1-dependent mechanisms of vascularization and vascular remodelling. Cardiovasc Res. 2010.

61. Brafman A, Mett I, Shafir M, Gottlieb H, Damari G, Gozlan-Kelner S, et al. Inhibition of oxygen-induced retinopathy in RTP801-deficient mice. Invest Ophthalmol Vis Sci. 2004;45(10):3796–805.

62. Tang Y, Scheef EA, Wang S, Sorenson CM, Marcus CB, Jefcoate CR, et al. CYP1B1 expression promotes the proangiogenic phenotype of endothelium through decreased intracellular oxidative stress and thrombospondin-2 expression. Blood. 2009;113(3): 744–54.

63. Caro AA, Cederbaum AI. Role of cytochrome P450 in phospholipase A2- and arachidonic acid-mediated cytotoxicity. Free Radic Biol Med. 2006;40(3):364–75.

64. Hardy P, Beauchamp M, Sennlaub F, Gobeil J, Tremblay L, Mwaikambo B, et al. New insights into the retinal circulation: inflammatory lipid mediators in ischemic retinopathy. Prostaglandins Leukot Essent Fat Acids. 2005;72(5):301–25.

65. Beauchamp MH, Sennlaub F, Speranza G, Gobeil J, Checchin D, Kermorvant-Duchemin E, et al. Redox-dependent effects of nitric oxide on microvascular integrity in oxygen-induced retinopathy. Free Radic Biol Med. 2004;37(11):1885–94.

66. Soghier LM, Brion LP. Cysteine, cystine or N-acetylcysteine supplementation in parenterally fed neonates. Cochrane Database Syst Rev. 2006 (4):CD004869. doi:10.1002/14651858.CD004869. pub2.

67. Brion LP, Bell EF, Raghuveer TS. Vitamin E supplementation for prevention of morbidity and mortality in preterm infants. Cochrane Database Syst Rev. 2003(4):CD003665. doi:10.1002/14651858. cd003665.

68. Dani C, Lori I, Favelli F, Frosini S, Messner H, Wanker P, et al. Lutein and zeaxanthin supplementation in preterm infants to prevent retinopathy of prematurity: a randomized controlled study. J Maternal-Fetal Neonatal Med. 2011;25(5):523–7.

69. Al Shabrawey M, Bartoli M, El Remessy AB, Ma G, Matragoon S, Lemtalsi T et al. Role of NADPH oxidase and Stat3 in statin-mediated protection against diabetic retinopathy. Invest Ophthalmol Vis Sci. 2008;49(7):3231–8.

70. Hoppe G, et al. Proc Natl Acad Sci U S A. 2016 May 3;113(18):E2516–25.

71. McCloskey M, Wang H, Jiang Y, Smith GW, Strange J, Hartnett ME. Anti-VEGF antibody leads to later atypical intravitreous neovascularization and activation of angiogenic pathways in a rat model of retinopathy of prematurity. Invest Ophthalmol Vis Sci. 2013;54(3):2020–6. doi:10.1167/iovs.13-11625.

72. Reynolds JD, Hardy RJ, Kennedy KA, Spencer R, van Heuven WAJ, Fielder AR. Lack of efficacy of light reduction in preventing retinopathy of prematurity. N Engl J Med. 1998;338:1572–6.

73. Rao S, Chun C, Fan J, Kofron JM, Yang MB, Hegde RS, et al. A direct and melanopsin-dependent fetal light response regulates mouse eye development. Nature. 2013;494(7436):243–6. doi:10.1038/nature11823.

74. Yang MB, Rao S, Copenhagen DR, Lang RA. Length of day during early gestation as a predictor of risk for severe retinopathy of prematurity. Ophthalmology. 2013;120(12):2706–13. doi:10.1016/j. ophtha.2013.07.051.

Classification of ROP

2

Thomas Lee

Keywords

Retinopathy of prematurity (ROP) · Threshold ROP · Plus disease · Neovascularization · Avascular retina

Retinopathy of prematurity (ROP) is an iatrogenic disease. Prior to 1940 it did not exist in humans and until 1941 no ophthalmologist had ever seen such case. That changed in 1940 when Dr. Martin Couney unveiled the country's first incubators for premature children that had pure oxygen to supplement the incubation chamber at the World's Fair in New York City. The following year, Dr. Theodore Terry in Boston, documented the first case of bilateral retrolental fibroplasia [1]. In the ensuing 10 years, it was estimated that approximately 7,000 premature babies in the United States went blind. It was not until 1986 that an international cooperative group formed and established the CRYO-ROP trial. The goal of the trial was to determine the natural history of this new disease and whether ablation of the avascular retina with cryotherapy would reduce the risk of blindness. To allow the international investigators to share data, the study established the International Classification of Retinopathy of Prematurity (ICROP). This system described the status of the disease based on three parameters: zone, stage, and presence of plus disease [2]. Taken together, these three measures determined whether a patient had mild ROP, pre-threshold ROP, or threshold ROP. This status would then determine the patient's schedule for follow-up as well as need for treatment.

Zone

Because the cardinal feature of ROP is the presence of avascular retina, the study created three zones that characterized where the normal retinal vasculature was present. The primary criterion for creating zones was that the physician would be able to make the determination based on indirect ophthalmoscopy alone (Fig. 2.1).

ZONE 1: Those children with the most posterior ROP where the normal retinal vessels had very little growth were termed Zone 1. Patients with Zone 1 had their retinal vessels extended from the optic nerve out to the periphery but not beyond the macula. To assist the examining ophthalmologist in determining whether a patient was in Zone 1, the study defined it as a circle centered at the optic nerve that had a radius twice the distance from the optic nerve to the fovea (Fig. 2.2a). To qualify as being in Zone 1, the examiner only needed to identify one clock hour where the retinal vessels stopped within the region. For a quick way to determine Zone 1, an examiner using a 28 diopter lens can place the edge of the lens to just encompass the optic nerve on one side of the image field. The other side of the lens would then be the edge of the Zone 1 (Fig. 2.2b). This technique is an easy way for the

T. Lee (✉)
Ophthalmology Department, The Vision Center, Children's Hospital Los Angeles, 4650 Sunset Blvd, MS 88, Los Angeles, CA 90027, USA
e-mail: ThLee@chla.usc.edu

© Springer International Publishing AG 2017
Andrés Kychenthal B. and Paola Dorta S. (eds.), *Retinopathy of Prematurity*,
DOI 10.1007/978-3-319-52190-9_2

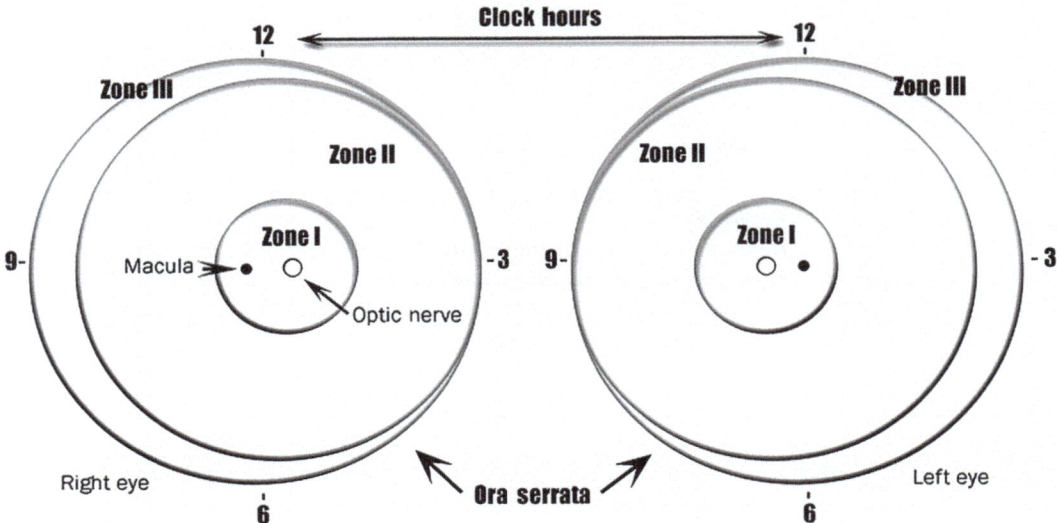

Fig. 2.1 ICROP exam form: standard form for documenting Zone and stage as well as presence of Plus disease

(a) **(b)**

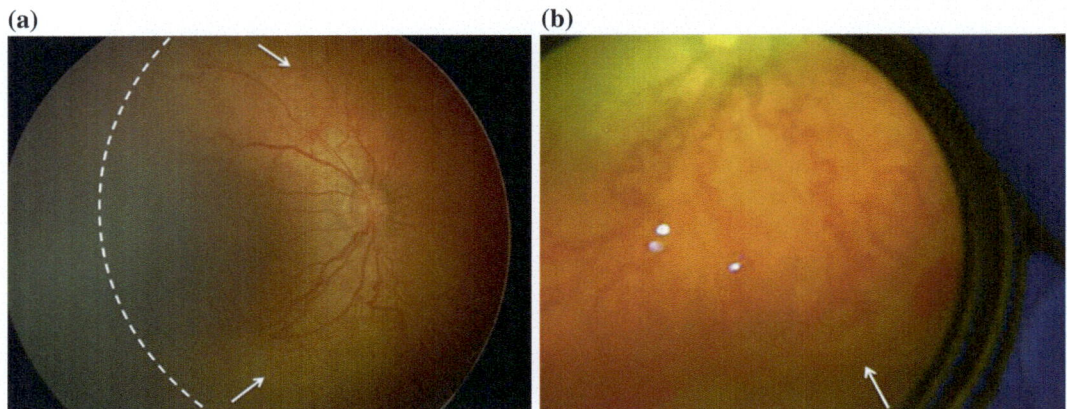

Fig. 2.2 a Example of Zone 1 ROP using a RetCam image. The *white dotted line* marks the edge of Zone 1. The *white arrows* show areas where the vascularized retina stops short of the Zone 1 border. **b** Example of Zone 1 ROP using a digital indirect ophthalmoscope and a 28 diopter lens where the optic nerve and the end of the vascularized retina (*white arrow*) can be seen in the same field of view

examiner to determine Zone 1 as long as the optic nerve is in view with a 28 diopter lens.

ZONE 2: This region is defined as retinal vessels that have extended past Zone 1 but remain within a larger circle that has a radius extending from the optic nerve to the nasal ora serrate (Fig. 2.3). From a practical standpoint, this would be an exam where the patient is not in Zone 1 but the retinal vessels do not extend all the way to the nasal ora serrata. Although the retinal vascular development usually has equal growth from the optic nerve in all directions, there are times that it can be asymmetric with the vessels extending all the way to the nasal ora serrata but falling temporally into Zone 2 in which case the patient would still be classified as Zone 2.

ZONE 3: This region is defined as the remaining retina beyond Zone 2 and mostly represents the most peripheral temporal retina. This

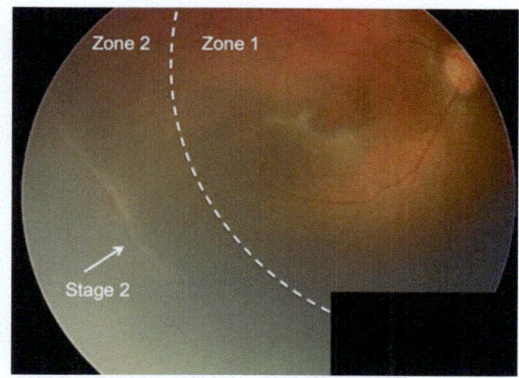

Fig. 2.3 Example of Zone 2 stage 2 ROP using a RetCam image. The vascularized retina extends beyond the border of Zone 1 (*white arrow*)

area can quickly identify when the retinal is fully vascularized nasally and the temporal aspect requires depression to visualize adequately.

Stage

Once the Zone has been identified, the next step is to determine the level of ROP at the interface between the vascular and avascular retina. Fundamentally the stage represents various levels of evolution of the pathologic angiogenesis. The neovascularization typically occurs at the edge of the vascularized retina. This neovascularization grows in a disorganized fashion that starts off as a white flat demarcation line. This is the very early phase of the process. As the pathologic neovascularization progresses, the vessels begin to accumulate at this location leading to an elevation/bump (some refer to the appearance of a "speed bump"). As the process continues the neovascularization begins to spill into the vitreous. This is the tipping point in the disease since the next phase is to recruit scar tissue along with the now vitreous involved vessels that can lead to a tractional detachment and blindness. To describe this, the CRYO-ROP study defined the different stages as follows:

Immature retina: when the retinal vessels stop and there is no visible demarcation line. This can be a challenge to identify because in the early exams there are often no clear landmarks to look for. Some people informally refer to this as stage 0 although this is not a terminology used by ICROP.

Stage 1: The retinal vessels stop and then a linear flat white line is present that usually runs the circumference of the vascular retina.

Stage 2: The neovascularization is now accumulating and has developed thickness that manifests as a linear bump (speed bump). Importantly, the neovascularization remains along the surface of the retina and is not beginning to extend off the retina into the cortical vitreous (Fig. 2.3).

Stage 3: The neovascularization has now been accumulated at the edge of the vascularized retina so that it is now extending into the vitreous. ICROP has called this extra retinal fibrosis proliferation. In cases of Zone 2 and Zone 3, this will at times be described as a sausage shaped stage 3. Unlike the white/pink color of stage 1 and 2, stage 3 will often have a red appearance consistent with the increased blood being shunted through the accumulating stage 3 (Fig. 2.4a, b). In more posterior Zone 1 disease, the stage 3 can appear as a direct extension of the normal retinal vessels but extending tangentially over the avascular retina. This is in contrast to the typical stage 3, which has the sausage-shaped appearance. Some refer to this as flat neovascularization [3].

Stage 4: As the stage 3 progresses to grow into the vitreous it can form a continuous sheet coming up from the edge of the vascularized retina. The appearance of a sheet/membrane is an ominous finding and often is a precursor to a cicatricial phase that can induce vitreous organization around the vascular sheet. This scar tissue can grow toward the vitreous base/posterior lens capsule resulting in traction, distortion, and

(a)   **(b)**

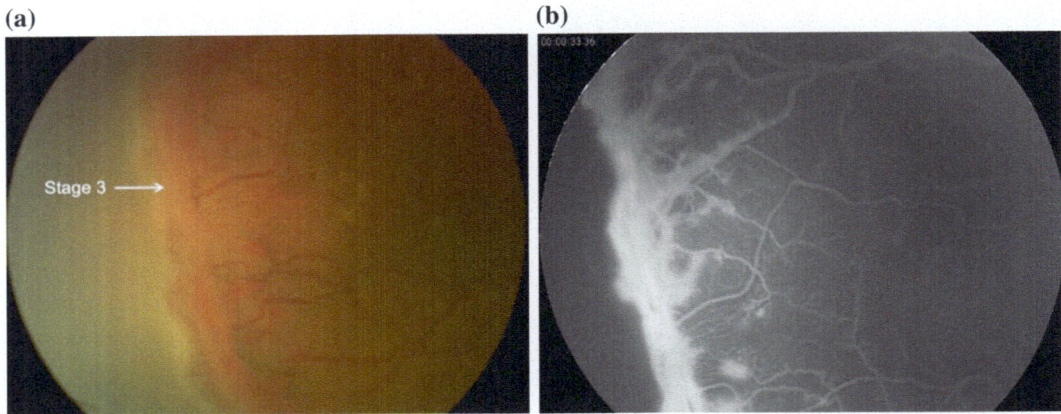

Fig. 2.4 a Stage 3 present temporally in the right eye (*white arrow*). **b** Fluorescein Angiography showing stage 3 at the edge of the vascularized retina

even detachment. Stage 4 occurs once the scar tissue causes enough traction to create a tractional detachment. Stage 4a describes a detachment that involves the peripheral retina that does not extend into the macula (Fig. 2.5). Stage 4b is when the traction extends more posteriorly and involves the macula itself. The detachment usually starts in the temporal periphery although can also involve the nasal retina as well. While stage 1–3 occurs prior to treatment, stage 4 can occur after treatment and may be accelerated by the absence

Fig. 2.5 Stage 4A detachment with an annular ring of fibrosis present tugging on the retina leading a tractional detachment

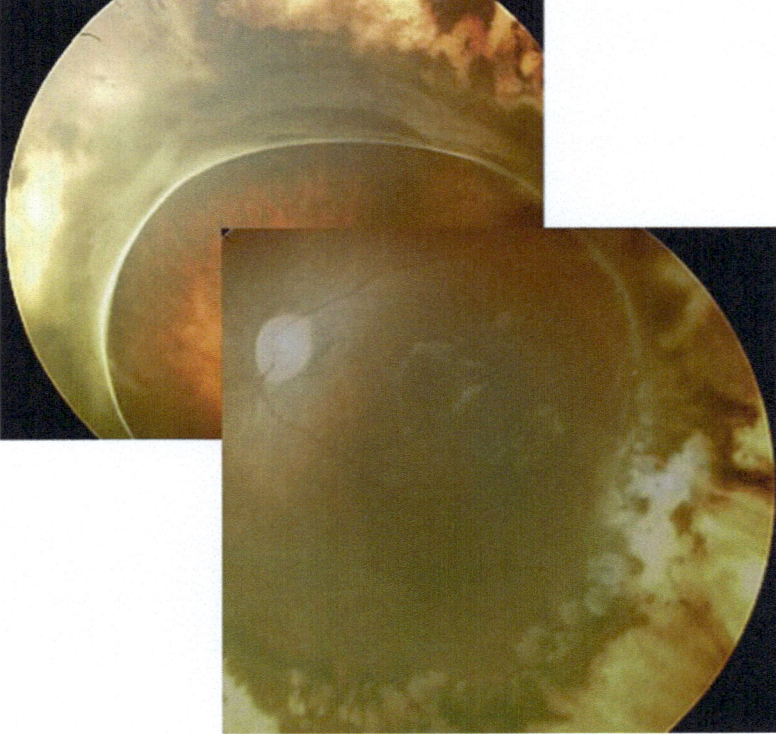

of vascular endothelial growth factor posttreatment leading to an accelerated cicatricial phase.

Stage 5: When stage 4 progresses, it can lead to a total retinal detachment termed stage 5. This is funnel detachment with generally traction in all four quadrants. Stage 5a refers to an open funnel while stage 5b refers to a closed funnel.

Plus Disease

ROP is characterized by progressive changes in the retinal vasculature. As the pathologic neo-vascularization progresses, it creates collateralization resulting in increased in blood flow. Clinically this is manifested as vascular dilation and tortuosity. At the beginning, these vascular changes are more apparent in the peripheral vessels adjacent to the shunt and may even precede the clinical detection of stage 3. As the stage 3 progresses, the peripheral dilation and tortuosity is sometimes described as arborization or decreased branching angle of the vessels. These vascular changes in the periphery can ultimately progress more posteriorly resulting in Plus disease. The CRYO-ROP study characterizes Plus Disease as dilation and tortuosity of the vessels exiting the optic nerve and involving at least six clock hours of the nerve (Fig. 2.6a). There was a standard photograph that was given as a reference (Fig. 2.6b). It is important to understand that the dilation and tortuosity of the peripheral vessels often seen with stage 3 do not constitute Plus Disease and that this term only refers to the nature of the vessels adjacent to the optic nerve.

The presence of Plus disease is now a key element in determining whether a patient qualifies for treatment. One fundamental problem with the definition is that it relies on the observer's own perception of what constitutes dilation and tortuosity. Studies have shown that even among experienced ROP examiners, there can be a wide variation on which exams qualify for Plus disease [4, 5]. There is also a modified term of Pre-plus disease, which is defined as vascular dilation and tortuosity that do not qualify as Plus disease [6].

Pre-threshold

One goal of the original CRYO-ROP Study was to identify eyes that would be at high risk of needing the treatment. These patients were identified as pre-threshold which included patients who were in Zone 1 (no Plus or stage 3)

(a)   (b)

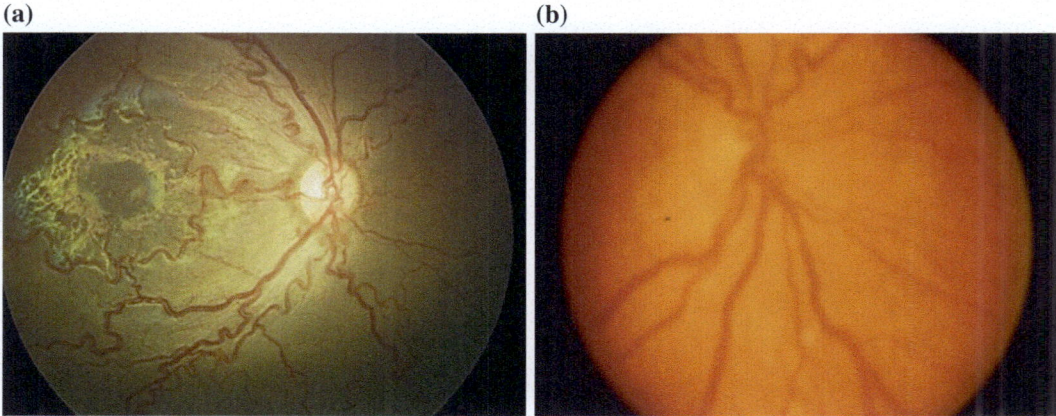

Fig. 2.6 **a** RetCam photography showing dilation and tortuosity of the posterior vessels as they exit the optic nerve. **b** Standard photograph showing Plus disease

or Zone 2 with Plus or stage 3 but not both. These children were placed on a more frequent examination schedule of at least every week or sooner as opposed to the recommended 2 week interval for patients with milder ROP.

Threshold

Threshold refers to an eye that has progressed beyond pre-threshold to include Zone 1 or Zone 2 with Plus disease and 5 continuous clock hours or 8 discontinuous clock hours of stage 3. In the CRYO-ROP study, patients with Threshold ROP received laser treatment or cryotherapy for avascular retina.

Early Treatment ROP Trial

Although patients with threshold ROP in Zone 2 did well, the Zone 1 patients still had a high failure rate and so a follow-up study, the Early Treatment for ROP (ETROP) trial [7–9], was started. This trial was designed to allow treatment earlier for those patients who were at a very high risk rather than waiting for full Threshold ROP. In this trial, pre-threshold was subdivided into Type 1 and Type 2. Type 2 was the milder form and included eyes in Zone 1 with no plus or stage 3 or eyes in Zone 2 with stage 3. Type 1 was any eye with Plus disease or a Zone 1 eye that developed stage 3. With this new criterion of Type 1 pre-threshold, the average time of laser treatment was now on average two weeks earlier and resulted in a reduction of the failure rate in Zone 1 disease.

References

1. Terry TL. Extreme prematurity and fibroplastic overgowth of persistent vascular sheath behind each crystal-line lens. I Preliminary report. Am J Ophthalmol. 1942;25:203–4.
2. The Committee for the Classification of Retinopathy of Prematurity. An international classification of retinopathy of prematurity. Arch Ophthalmol. 1984;102(8):1130–4.
3. Vinekar A, Trese MT, Capone A. Jr. Photographic screening for retinopathy of prematurity (PHOTO-ROP) cooperative group. Evolution of retinal detachment in posterior retinopathy of prematurity: Impact on treatment approach. Am J Ophthalmol. 2008;145(3):548–55.
4. Chiang MF, Jiang L, Gelman R, Du YE, Flynn JT. Interexpert agreement of plus disease diagnosis in retinopathy of prematurity. Arch Ophthalmol. 2007;125(7):875–80.
5. Slidsborg C, Forman JL, Fielder AR, Crafoord S, Baggesen K, Bangsgaard R, Fledelius HC, Greisen G, la Cour M. Experts do not agree when to treat retinopathy of prematurity based on plus disease. Br J Ophthalmol. 2012;96(4):549–53.
6. International Committee for the Classification of Retinopathy of Prematurity. The international classification of retinopathy of prematurity revisited. Arch Ophthalmol. 2005;123(7):991–9.
7. Early Treatment For Retinopathy Of Prematurity Cooperative Group. Revised indications for the treatment of retinopathy of prematurity: results of the early treatment for retinopathy of prematurity randomized trial. Arch Ophthalmol. 2003;121(12):1684–94.
8. Hardy RJ, Good WV, Dobson V, Palmer EA, Phelps DL, Quintos M, Tung B. Early treatment for retinopathy of prematurity cooperative group. multicenter trial of early treatment for retinopathy of prematurity: Study design. Control Clin Trials. 2004;25(3):311–25.
9. Good WV. Early treatment for retinopathy of prematurity, cooperative group. Final results of the Early Treatment for Retinopathy of Prematurity (ETROP) randomized trial. Trans Am Ophthalmol Soc. 2004;102:233–48.

Retinopathy of Prematurity Screening—Current and Future Considerations

Clare M. Wilson, Anna L. Ells and Alistair R. Fielder

Keywords

Retinopathy of prematurity (ROP) · Screening guidelines · Telemedicine · Screening · RetCam · Sight-threatening ROP

Introduction

Screening for retinopathy of prematurity (ROP) and the optimum treatment of severe disease in order to prevent blindness requires detailed understanding of the infants at risk and timely eye examinations. Many practical screening challenges secondary to the diversity of disease exist. These issues fall into two main categories—First, which infants should be screened? And second, how should the infants be screened? The diversity of ROP presentation is exemplified in its geographical distribution, with variations in those infants at risk for severe ROP and altered temporal development of disease in different locations. The risk of ROP is ubiquitous amongst the premature neonatal population; the only countries fortunate to be exempt from the

condition are those paradoxically unfortunately unable to provide survival care for their preterm infants. In high-income countries in the late 1950s, the first epidemic of ROP occurred in relatively high birth weight (BW) and gestational age (GA) babies as they were treated with high oxygen concentrations within the neonatal intensive care units (NICUs), as the associated dangers of oxygen to the eye were not realized. Unfortunately, in many low- and middle-income countries today supplemental oxygen levels are not monitored, leading to the manifestation of ROP in similarly high GA, high BW infants in these countries, as in the first epidemic [1]. Despite numerous screening guidelines not all populations and situations are adequately covered, so preventable visual loss from ROP still occurs. This chapter will present and discuss screening guidelines and challenges to successful implementation of these guidelines. Evidence-based guidelines are very important for global ROP screening but also manpower for ROP services are in great demand in many parts of the world. Potential solutions to these problems include algorithms linked to the increase in weight of preterm infants over time, which may decrease the number of infants requiring an eye exam and a telemedicine approach to ROP with automated analysis of image characteristics on site.

C.M. Wilson (✉)
Ophthalmology, Chelsea and Westminster,
369 Fulham Road, London SW10 9NH, UK
e-mail: clarewil25@yahoo.com

A.L. Ells
Department of Surgery, University of Calgary,
5340 1st Street SW, Calgary, AB T2H OV8, Canada
e-mail: annaells@mae.com

A.R. Fielder
Optometry & Visual Science, City University
London, Northampton Square,
London EC1V 0HB, UK
e-mail: a.fielder@city.ac.uk

© Springer International Publishing AG 2017
Andrés Kychenthal B. and Paola Dorta S. (eds.), *Retinopathy of Prematurity*,
DOI 10.1007/978-3-319-52190-9_3

Screening Guidelines

It was first reported in 1988 that treatment for severe ROP improved visual outcomes and this made ROP screening and treatment a priority [2]. In the UK, for instance, in the early 1980s, less than 10 ophthalmologists were involved in ROP screening, but by 1995, 183 ophthalmologists screened for ROP in 96% units in the UK caring for preterm [3]. ROP screening is included in the Action Plan 2006–2011 in *"Vision 2020 The Right to Sight Global Initiative for the Elimination of Avoidable Blindness"* with the overall aim to provide services to treat children with ROP and with three specific strategies: first, "examine premature infants at risk of ROP, treat those with severe disease and promote oxygen monitoring"; Second, ensure availability of ophthalmologists experienced in indirect ophthalmoscopy to identify premature infants in intensive neonatal

care who require treatment for ROP"; Third, "ensure that infants at risk have fundus examinations starting at 4–6 weeks after birth and that infants with severe disease are treated immediately by laser or cryotherapy." [4].

Many countries have created ROP screening guidelines [5]. Table 3.1 includes a selection of these. We will use the frequently used terms low-, middle-, and high-income countries, but we emphasize that this does not always precisely equate to the quality of care in every neonatal intensive care unit (NICU) in a particular country. In high-income countries, such as the USA and UK, the standard of neonatal care is high and while there will be variations, these will probably be relatively minor compared to other countries such as India, South Africa, and Brazil where the standard of care may vary widely between individual NICUs, even in one city, from the highest standard in well-resourced units to those with

Table 3.1 A global selection of screening criteria

Country	GA (weeks) and BW (g)	Notes
Argentina [74]	≤32 weeks and/or 1500 g	Include also 1500–2000 g with unstable clinical course, predisposing factors or prolonged oxygen therapy
Brazil [16]	≤32 weeks and/or ≤1500 g	Include also larger and more mature babies with illnesses and other risk factors, e.g. sepsis, respiratory problems, multiple births
Canada [73]	<31 weeks and <1251 g	Include also babies 1251–2000 g if at high risk due to complex clinical course
Chile [75]	<33 weeks and <1500 g	Include also babies between 1500 and 2000 g with unstable clinical course, predisposing risk factor or prolonged oxygen therapy
Colombia [77]	≤32 weeks and/or ≤1800 g	Include also >1800 g with unstable clinical course, predisposing factors or prolonged oxygen therapy
Mexico [76]	≤34 weeks and/or ≤1750 g	
Sweden [23]	<31 weeks	Include also larger babies severely ill
India [17]	<34 weeks and/or <1750 g	Include also babies 34–36 weeks or 1750–2000 g if there are risk factors
UK [7]	<31 weeks or <1251 g one criterion to be met	Must be screened. No additional sickness criteria
UK [7]	31 to <32 weeks or 1251–1501 g one criterion to be met	Should be screened
USA [42]	≤30 weeks or <1500 g	Include also "selected" 1500–2000 g or >30 weeks if unstable clinical course with cardiorespiratory support and at high risk
South Africa [78]	<30 weeks and <1500 g	Also selected 1500–2000 g if risk factors or oxygen monitoring suboptimal—includes guidance on oxygen monitoring

sparse resources in which unblended oxygen is administered. For example, Zin et al. mention that in Rio de Janeiro the better NICUs could employ narrower guidelines compared to other units in the same city [6].

Which Infants Need to be Screened?

High-Income Countries

In high-income countries, with a relatively uniform high level of neonatal care, most have devised inclusion criteria, based on gestational age, birth weight alone or with sickness criteria. There is very little data on the specificity of illness factors which are risk factors for ROP [7]. It is pertinent to note that in high-income countries with excellent neonatal care, inappropriately excessive oxygen administration is rare (not denying the importance of oxygen in ROP pathogenesis) and the additional risk factors are likely to be sepsis, transfusions, general sickness, and prolonged cardiorespiratory support—which are most probably nonspecific indicators of illness. Almost all ROP requiring treatment affects babies <31 weeks GA or <1250 g BW, but it does occasionally occur in larger and more mature babies [7–9]. More data is required to determine whether the safest, most effective, and efficient method to include the outliers is by raising the GA and BW bar and disregarding a sickness score, or by setting lower level limits and combining GA and BW with a "sickness" criterion which will robustly identify the larger infant.

Low- and Middle-Income Countries

In low- and middle-income countries, with variations in the standard of neonatal care, larger and more mature infants are at risk of developing sight-threatening ROP [1, 10–13] compared with those in high-income countries. Recent publications from India illustrate the issue with infants <36 weeks GA and >2500 g BW requiring treatment [13–15]. Clearly basing inclusion criteria on GA and BW alone under these circumstances would be quite inappropriate as many babies would be unnecessarily screened and the manpower demand for screening simply could not be met. Thus in these communities a sickness criterion needs to be included for those larger and more mature babies without the GA and BW but who are at risk of sight-threatening ROP as screened.

As well, in many instances, the GA may not be known. As indicated in Table 3.1 the GA and BW inclusion criteria are wider in those middle-income countries which have guidelines such as Brazil [16] and India [17]. Inappropriate excessive oxygen administration—sometimes unblended—has long been suspected to be a risk factor. Shah et al. reported a high incidence of aggressive posterior ROP (APROP) in babies <35 weeks GA who had received unblended oxygen and that following crude oxygen blending this incidence fell dramatically [14].

Clinical management within the NICU's is continually changing, so reevaluation of evidence-based inclusion criteria for infants requiring a screening eye exam will be necessary from time to time.

When to Screen?

ROP Natural History

An effective and efficient screening program requires understanding of the natural history of ROP. This has been studied in population-based [18–20] and treatment studies [21–23]. Findings have been very consistent over the 20-year period in high-income countries, showing that the onset and progression of ROP are governed predominantly by postmenstrual and not postnatal age, although there is a slight acceleration of the process in the most immature infants [20]. The rate of progress through the stages is approximately one stage per 7–10 days: thus in the Early Treatment of Retinopathy of Prematurity Study (ETROP) the median age for stages 1, 2, and 3 and plus disease was 34.1, 35.1, 36.6, and 36.0 weeks post menstrual age (PMA), respectively [24]. ROP very rarely requires treatment before 31 weeks PMA and the mean age for treatment of Type I (prethreshold) and threshold disease in ETROP was 35.2 weeks PMA (range 30.6–42.1 weeks) and 37.0 weeks PMA (range 31.9–46.6 weeks) essentially identical to previous studies [25].

With respect to middle- and low-income countries and larger infants, Carden et al. reported on 100 preterm infants <1900 g BW and <35 weeks GA in Vietnam who required treatment for threshold ROP at 36.25 weeks PMA (range 31.4–44.3 weeks) [11]. From India, Shah et al. reported on laser treatment to 93 babies (<2250 g BW and <35 weeks GA) at mean age of 37 weeks PMA (range 30–40 weeks), while Jalali et al. (2011) treated 115 babies with APROP at a mean age of 34.6 weeks PMA (range 31–51 weeks PMA) [14, 15]. Thus, information to date confirms that the natural history of ROP is governed by postmenstrual age so that the mean age of infants requiring treatment at threshold ROP is approximately 37 weeks and at Type I prethreshold around 35 weeks even in larger infants. Progression through the stages of disease will be compressed in the larger infants and the National Neonatology Foundation of India guideline recommends screening by 2–3 weeks of age [17].

When to Start Screening?

Screening should commence before ROP requires treatment (Table 3.2). Several ROP guidelines have given a single postnatal age for the commencement of screening examinations, e.g., 6–7 weeks for the 1995 UK guideline [3] and 4–6 weeks in the Vision 2020 Action Plan [4]. While this had the merit of simplicity, it did not take into consideration the natural history of ROP and consequently required excessive examinations of the most immature infants and yet would have missed the opportunity for treatment in the largest and most mature infant. Several national guidelines have now followed the approach suggested by Reynolds et al. in which the commencement of screening is tailored to the infant's GA [26]. This is shown in Table 3.2 and has been extended by authors beyond 32 weeks for the purpose of this article. It is important to note that larger birth weight infants should have earlier screening exams.

When Screening Can Be Safely Terminated

The decision to terminate screening safely is critical and depends on whether or not the infant

Table 3.2 Suggested age for first screening examination

Gestational age (weeks)	Age at first ROP screening examination	
	Postnatal Age (weeks)	Postmenstrual age (weeks)
22	8	30
23	7	30
24	6	30
25	5	30
26	4	30
27	4	31
28	4	32
29	4	33
30	4	34
31	4	35
32	3	35
33	2	35
34	2	36
35	2	37

had any ROP. In those infants not ever having had any ROP, most guidelines recommend that eye exams should continue until there is adequate retinal vascularization to zone III and not to stop screening before 37 weeks of PMA. Infants that have had ROP throughout their clinical course require at least two examinations with signs of regression of ROP.

Telemedicine Approach to ROP

Telemedicine refers to the use of information technologies to support health care between participants who are separated from each other. It may be a possible solution to some of the screening challenges in the management of ROP.

Over the last 15 years, research studies using a telemedicine approach to ROP screening have consistently demonstrated the ability to identify infants at risk for severe ROP needing treatment. There are over 35 peer-reviewed published studies that document feasibility and accuracy of this approach [27–31]. Advances in imaging techniques have enabled the manufacture of digital cameras specifically for imaging the posterior segment and retina of the premature infants. The RetCam digital camera system (Clarity Medical Systems, Pleasanton, California, USA) is the most commonly used camera for neonatal ophthalmic imaging. The wide-angle lens gives a panoramic view of the retina, and the capture and save feature enables photographic documentation of retinal pathology which may become part of the permanent medical record in addition to its use in telemedicine. Retinal photographic documentation of infants at risk for ROP using the RetCam camera with remote interpretation of digital images has been favorably assessed in many studies. Recently, a large multicenter study published results that support the validity of remote evaluation by trained nonphysician readers of digital retinal images taken by trained nonphysician imagers from infants at risk for severe ROP [32–34].

Several telemedicine studies have documented identification of severe ROP disease one to two weeks earlier than the clinical binocular

indirect ophthalmoscopy (BIO) standard [35, 36]. Earlier identification of disease leads to earlier treatment of severe ROP and early treatment results in better visual outcomes [37–39]. This is consistent with major clinical trials in diabetic retinopathy that document the efficacy of digital imaging with remote evaluation as better than ophthalmologists' exams in detecting the features of diabetic retinopathy [40, 41]. The use of telemedicine to manage infants with ROP offers the potential to address the shortage of physician expertise, standardize, and improve the quality of ROP evaluations and optimize the timing of treatment of premature infants.

An Ophthalmic Technology Assessment report commissioned by the American Academy of Ophthalmology has evaluated the accuracy of detecting clinically significant ROP using wide-angle digital retinal photography from the literature currently available [42]. It reviewed seven level I papers and three level III papers. Of these ten papers, seven of them reported a high sensitivity and specificity for detecting ROP needing treatment using digital imaging.

Chiang et al. reported on multiple "Real-World ROP Management Programs" [43]. These programs have successfully set up ROP telemedicine programs and have published data supporting their validity. The largest published dataset of infants screened for ROP using telemedicine is from Bangalore, India. This telemedicine program, KIDROP (Karnataka Internet Assisted Diagnosis of Retinopathy of Prematurity), has been screening in remote neonatal intensive care units (NICU's) in rural regions where ROP screening does not exist [44–47]. Trained and certified technicians visit multiple hospitals on a fixed schedule in many districts of Karnataka state (inhabited by 64 million people), and using the Retcam Shuttle, image infants who are either resident to that NICU or referred to the program. Images are stored, analyzed, and uploaded on a secure Tele-ROP platform (i2i Tele-solutions Ltd, Bangalore, India) for the expert to view and report on a smart phone, tablet or computer, in real-time, using a standardized template [17, 45]. In Germany, Lorenz et al. showed 100%

detection of suspected ROP treatment warranted cases in a prospective study [48]. In the USA, the Stanford University Network for Diagnosis of ROP has reported a 100% sensitivity and 90% specificity at detecting treatment warranted cases of ROP [49]. The Joint Technical Report on "Telemedicine for Evaluation of Retinopathy of Prematurity" recently published by the American Academy of Pediatrics Section on Ophthalmology, American Academy of Ophthalmology, and American Association of Certified Orthoptists also reinforces the important impact of telemedicine in the future management of ROP [50].

Future Technology of ROP Screening

Less than 10% of neonates screened for ROP will require treatment, so the vast majority either do not develop ROP or it is mild and self-limited. This offers two options for screening: identifying the eye not at risk of developing sight-threatening ROP or predicting reliably the eye which is likely to progress. Predictive factors for likelihood of disease progression can be reliably isolated. Predictive factors for ROP progression studied thus far include post natal weight gain, serum IGF-1 levels and quantifiable vessel changes in the retina. The dichotomous distinction between disease presence and disease absence may be a warranted first step in assessing these infants. There is also growing evidence that genetic factors are linked with disease severity, and in the more distant future, genetic screening may also add to the decision-making process of which babies are more likely to benefit from eye screening examinations.

An alternative and complementary approach to identifying either the eye with no/mild or severe ROP is through retinal vessel analysis. Image analysis techniques have progressed rapidly, and over the last decade retinal vessel analysis tools have been developed specifically to assess the vascular changes in the posterior pole associated with plus disease of ROP. Image segmentation isolates areas of interest within an image. There are many different image segmentation techniques and these can broadly be divided into ridge-based and region-based techniques. These techniques have been applied to retinal images by many teams globally to identify blood vessels in images. Locating the tiniest blood vessels in preterm neonates has been challenging for software, but progress is being made and the accuracy of these systems may consequently equip them to be the most sensitive and specific tools for finding features in adult images. The first reports of semi-automated image analysis techniques for identifying and then quantifying retinal vessels from RetCam images were from Imperial College London where Retinal Image multiScale Analysis (RISA) had been developed [51].

RISA has been used to quantify arterial tortuosity in ROP and subsequently showed that in plus disease arteriolar and venous curvature, diameter and tortuosity index are all increased compared to those without plus disease [52]. The rate of change in venous parameters has been correlated with plus disease development using RISA, with the highest area under the curve reported in venous tortuosity index for weekly rate of change [53]. Additional computer-assisted vessel detection software has been developed, including, ROPtool, developed at Duke University, USA [54, 55] and Computer-Aided Image Analysis of the Retina (CAIAR), developed from RISA to enable quicker image analysis due to more accurate image segmentation techniques [56–58].

These semi-automated systems can detect plus disease of ROP with comparable or even better accuracy to experts [58–61]. As well as vessel width and tortuosity, other retinal parameters such as vessel branching pattern and arcade angles may add strength to automated digital image analysis as a screening tool for ROP [62–65].

Currently, there are limitations to automated image analysis—while tortuosity can be accurately calculated, width measurements are less robust and all methods are slow. The difficulty for man and machine to distinguish arterioles from venules maybe an unnecessary concern, as we have recently shown that the four most tortuous vessels in an image, regardless of their vessel type, are correlated well with treated versus not treated eyes [66]. With improved retinal image segmentation methods, mathematical combinations of individual feature values such as width and tortuosity, replication of work using larger datasets, and multidisciplinary collaborative efforts, these efforts will surely be worthwhile. Research is working toward more accurate, faster, and completely automated on-site software that quantifies plus disease and morphological features of those eyes requiring treatment for severe ROP.

WINROP (Weight, IGF-1 levels, Neonatal, ROP) is a surveillance algorithm developed by Lofqvist and colleagues in Sweden [67]. It measures weekly IGF-1 levels and weekly weight from birth until 36 weeks. It correctly identified all babies subsequently requiring laser treatment for proliferative ROP and also all infants with low risk ROP in a group of 50 preterm infants [67]. A further study of 354 infants in Sweden using only postnatal weight gain showed a 100% sensitivity and 84.5% specificity [68] and this was validated in a US cohort of 318 infants, again accurately predicting all babies who went on to develop ROP requiring treatment [69]. Binenbaum et al. reported a predictive model based on postnatal weight gain that may reduce the need for ROP screening [70].

There is growing evidence that genetic susceptibility plays a role in development of severe ROP. Three genes encoding for the Wnt and Norrin signaling pathways have been described to cause familial exudative vitreoretinopathy (FEVR), and two of these have been identified in infants developing ROP. These are the NDP gene (X-linked FEVR) and the FZD4 (autosomal dominant FEVR). Ells et al. identified two novel mutations (Ala370Gly and Lys203Asn) in the FZD4 gene in 2 infants out of 71 infants with severe ROP [71]. This mutation was not found in the 33 infants in the mild to no ROP group, or in 173 random Caucasian samples. Mutation in the NDP gene has been calculated to account for 3% of cases of severe ROP [72].

In summary, many evidence-based screening guidelines, developed by each country, have emerged in the last two decades, and have

increased our ability to identify those infants at greatest risk for ROP requiring treatment. Challenges to providing the screening examinations by on-site ophthalmologists have been balanced by innovative research for possible solutions. These include telemedicine programs, quantitative image analysis, and awareness of genetic vulnerabilities and weight gain algorithms. These new and future screening methods are complementary and may facilitate the development of a nonphysician screening in which approximately 90% of infants, who will never develop severe ROP, can be identified. Only those infants close to developing sight-threatening ROP will then be required to be examined by an ophthalmologist. This could be a timely and cost-effective way of providing screening in low-, middle-, and high-income countries.

References

1. Gilbert C. Retinopathy of prematurity: a global perspective of the epidemics: population of babies at risk and implications for control. Early Hum Dev. 2008;84:77–82.
2. Cryotherapy for Retinopathy of Prematurity Cooperative Group. Multicentre trial of cryotherapy for retinopathy of prematurity: preliminary results. Arch Ophthalmol. 1988;106:471–9.
3. Haines L, Fielder AR, Scrivener R, et al. Retinopathy of prematurity in the UK I: the organisation of services for screening and treatment. Eye (Lond). 2002;16:33–8.
4. Vision 2020: The Right to Sight. Action Plan 2006–2011; IAPB, Vision 2020, WHO. www.who.int/blindness/Vision2020_report.
5. Ells A, Hicks M, Fielden M, et al. Severe retinopathy of prematurity: longitudinal observation of disease and screening implications. Eye (Lond). 2005;19:138–44.
6. Zin AA, Moreira ME, Bunce C, et al. Retinopathy of prematurity in 7 neonatal units in Rio de Janeiro: screening criteria and workload implications. Pediatrics. 2010;126:e410–7.
7. Wilkinson AR, Haines L, Head K, et al. UK retinopathy of prematurity guideline. Early Hum Dev 2008;84:71–4. Guideline in full @ www.rcpch.ac.uk and www.rcophth.ac.uk.
8. Hutchinson AK, O'Neil JW, Morgan EN, et al. Retinopathy of prematurity in infants with birth weights greater than 1250 g. J AAPOS. 2003;7:190–4.
9. Yanovitch TL, Siatkowski RM, McCaffree M, et al. Retinopathy of prematurity in infants with birth

weight > or = 1250 grams-incidence, severity, and screening guideline cost-analysis. J AAPOS. 2006;10:128–34.

10. Gilbert C, Fielder A, Gordillo L, et al. International NO-ROP Group. Characteristics of infants with severe retinopathy of prematurity in countries with low, moderate, and high levels of development: implications for screening programs. Pediatrics. 2005;115:e518–25.

11. Carden SM, Luu LN, Nguyen TX, et al. Retinopathy of prematurity: postmenstrual age at threshold in a transitional economy is similar to that in developed countries. Clin Exp Ophthalmol. 2008;36:159–61.

12. Chen Y, Li X. Characteristics of severe retinopathy patients in China: a repeat of the first epidemic? Br J Ophthalmol. 2006;90:268–71.

13. Vinekar A, Dogra MR, Sangtam T, et al. Retinopathy of prematurity in Asian Indian babies weighing greater than 1250 grams at birth: ten year data from a tertiary care center in a developing country. Indian J Ophthalmol. 2007;55:331–6.

14. Shah PK, Narendran V, Kalpana N. Aggressive posterior retinopathy of prematurity in large preterm babies in South India. Arch Dis Child Fetal Neonatal Ed. 2012;97:F371–5.

15. Jalali S, Kesarwani S, Hussain A. Outcomes of a protocol-based management for zone I retinopathy of prematurity: The Indian twin cities screening program report number 2. Am J Ophthalmol. 2011;151:719–24.

16. Zin A, Florêncio T, Fortes Filho JB et al. Brazilian society of pediatrics, brazilian council of ophthalmology and brazilian society of pediatric ophthalmology. Brazilian guidelines proposal for screening and treatment of retinopathy of prematurity (ROP). Arq Bras Oftalmol 2007;70:875–83.

17. Pejaver RK, Vinekar A, Bilagi A. National Neonatology foundation's evidence based clinical practice guidelines 2010. Retinopathy of Prematurity (NNF India, Guidelines) 2010;253–62.

18. Fielder AR, Shaw DE, Robinson J, et al. Natural history of retinopathy of prematurity: a prospective study. Eye. 1992;6:233–42.

19. Holmström G, el Azazi M, Jacobson L and Lennerstrand G. A population based, prospective study of the development of ROP in prematurely born children in the Stockholm area of Sweden. Br J Ophthalmol 1993;77:417–23.

20. Austeng D, Källen KB, Hellström A, Tornqvist K, Holmström GE. Natural history of retinopathy of prematurity in infants born before 27 weeks' gestation in Sweden. Arch Ophthalmol. 2010;128:1289–94.

21. Palmer EA, Flynn JT, Hardy RJ, et al. The cryotherapy for retinopathy of prematurity cooperative group. Incidence and early course of retinopathy of prematurity. Ophthalmology. 1991;98:1628–40.

22. Reynolds JD, Dobson V, Quinn GE et al. on behalf of the CRYO-ROP and LIGHT-ROP Cooperative Groups. Evidence-based screening criteria for retinopathy of prematurity: natural history data from CRYO-ROP and LIGHT-ROP Studies. Arch Ophthalmol 2002;120:1470–6.

23. Holmström GE, Hellström A, Jakobsson PG, et al. Swedish national register for retinopathy of prematurity (SWEDROP) and the evaluation of screening in Sweden. Arch Ophthalmol. 2012;130:1418–24.

24. Good WV, Hardy RJ, Dobson V, et al. Early Treatment for Retinopathy of Prematurity Cooperative Group. The incidence and course of retinopathy of prematurity: findings from the early treatment for retinopathy of prematurity study. Pediatrics. 2005;116:15–23.

25. Good WV. Final results of the early treatment for retinopathy of prematurity (ETROP) randomized trial. Trans Am Ophthalmol Soc. 2004;102:233–50.

26. Reynolds JD. Malpractice and the quality of care in retinopathy of prematurity (an American Ophthalmological Society thesis). Trans Am Ophthalmol Soc. 2007;105:461–80.

27. Chiang MF, Wang L, Busuioc M, et al. Telemedical retinopathy of prematurity diagnosis: Accuracy, reliability, and image quality. Arch Ophthalmol. 2007;125(11):1531–8.

28. Silva RA, Murakami Y, Jain A, et al. Stanford university network for diagnosis of retinopathy of prematurity (SUNDROP): 18-month experience with telemedicine screening. Graefes Arch Clin Exp Ophthalmol. 2009;247(1):129–36.

29. Wu C, Petersen RA, VanderVeen DK. RetCam imaging for retinopathy of prematurity screening. J AAPOS. 2006;10(2):107–11.

30. Telemedicine approaches to evaluating acute-phase retinopathy of prematurity: study design. Graham E Quinn; e-ROP Cooperative Group. Ophthalmic Epidemiol. 2014;21(4):256–67.

31. Weaver DT, Murdock TJ. Telemedicine detection of type 1 ROP in a distant neonatal intensive care unit. J AAPOS. 2012;16(3):229–33.

32. Daniel E, Quinn GE, Hildebrand PL, Ells A, Hubbard GB 3rd, Capone A Jr, Martin ER, Ostroff CP, Smith E, Pistilli M, Ying GS; e-ROP Cooperative Group. Validated system for centralized grading of retinopathy of prematurity: telemedicine approaches to evaluating acute-phase retinopathy of prematurity (e-ROP) Study. JAMA Ophthalmol. 2015 Mar 26.

33. Ying GS, Quinn GE, Wade KC, Repka MX, Baumritter A, Daniel E; e-ROP Cooperative Group. Predictors for the development of referral-warranted retinopathy of prematurity in the telemedicine approaches to evaluating acute-phase retinopathy of prematurity (e-ROP) study. JAMA Ophthalmol. 20151;133(3):304–11.

34. Quinn GE, Ying GS, Daniel E, Hildebrand PL, Ells A, Baumritter A, Kemper AR, Schron EB, Wade K; e-ROP Cooperative Group. Validity of a telemedicine system for the evaluation of acute-phase retinopathy of prematurity. JAMA Ophthalmol. 2014;132(10):1178–84.

35. Ells AL, Holmes JM, Astle WF, et al. Telemedicine approach to screening for severe retinopathy of prematurity: A pilot study. Ophthalmology. 2003;110(11):2113–7.

36. Photographic Screening for Retinopathy of Prematurity (Photo-ROP) Cooperative Group. The photographic screening for retinopathy of prematurity study (photo-ROP) primary outcomes. Retina 2008;28(3 Suppl):S47–54.

37. Good WV. Early Treatment for Retinopathy of Prematurity Cooperative Group. The early treatment for retinopathy of prematurity study: Structural findings at age 2 years. Br J Ophthalmol. 2006;90 (11):1378–82.

38. Hardy RJ, Good WV, Dobson V, et al. The early treatment for retinopathy of prematurity clinical trial: Presentation by subgroups versus analysis within subgroups. Br J Ophthalmol. 2006;90(11):1341–2.

39. Fransen SR, Leonard-Martin TC, Feuer WJ, et al. Clinical evaluation of patients with diabetic retinopathy: Accuracy of the inoveon diabetic retinopathy-3DT system. Ophthalmology. 2002;109(3):595–601.

40. Lee P. Telemedicine: Opportunities and challenges for the remote care of diabetic retinopathy. Arch Ophthalmol. 1999;117(12):1639–40.

41. Good WV, Hardy RJ, Dobson V et al. The incidence and course of retinopathy of prematurity: Findings from the early treatment for retinopathy of prematurity study. Pediatrics. 2005;116(1):15–23 (Early Hum Dev 1996;46:239–58).

42. American Academy of Pediatrics. Section on Ophthalmology. American academy of ophthalmology, American association for pediatric ophthalmology and strabismus, American association of certified orthoptists. Screening examination of premature infants for retinopathy of prematurity. Pediatrics. 2013;131:189–95.

43. Chiang MF, Melia M, Buffenn AN, et al. Detection of clinically significant retinopathy of prematurity using wide-angle digital retinal photography. Ophthalmology. 2012;119:1272–80.

44. Vinekar A, Avadhani K, Braganza S, et al. Outcomes of a protocol-based management for zone 1 retinopathy of prematurity: the Indian Twin Cities ROP Screening Program report number 2. Am J Ophthalmol. 2011;152(4):712.

45. Vinekar A. IT-enabled innovation to prevent infant blindness in rural India: The KIDROP experience. J Indian Bus Res. 2011;3(2):98–102.

46. Vinekar A, Jayadev C, Bauer N. Need for telemedicine in retinopathy of prematurity in middle-income countries: e-ROP versus KIDROP. JAMA Ophthalmol. 2015;133(3):360–1.

47. Vinekar A, Gilbert C, Dogra M, Kurian M, Shainesh G, Shetty B, Bauer N. The KIDROP model of combining strategies for providing retinopathy of prematurity screening in underserved areas in India using wide-field imaging, tele-medicine, non-physician graders and smart phone reporting. Indian J Ophthalmol. 2014;62(1):41–9.

48. Lorenz B, Spasovska K, Elflein H, Schneider N. Wide-field digital imaging based telemedicine for screening for acute retinopathy of prematurity (ROP): six-year results of a multicentre field study. Graefes Arch Clin Exp Ophthalmol. 2009;247:1251–62.

49. Murakami Y, Silva RA, Jain A, et al. Stanford university network for diagnosis of retinopathy of prematurity (SUNDROP): 18-month experience with telemedicine screening. Graefes Arch Clin Exp Ophthalmol. 2009;247:129–36.

50. Fierson WM, Capone A Jr. American academy of pediatrics section on ophthalmology; american academy of ophthalmology, American association of certified orthoptists. Report of a joint working party. Retinopathy of prematurity: guidelines for screening and treatment. Royal College of Ophthalmologists and British Association of Perinatal Medicine. Telemedicine for evaluation of retinopathy of prematurity. Pediatrics. 2015;135(1):e238–54.

51. Swanson C, Coker KD, Parker KH, Moseley MJ, Fielder AR. Semiautomated computer analysis of vessel growth in preterm infants without and with retinopathy of prematurity. Br J Ophthalmol. 2003;87(12):1474–7.

52. Gelman R, Martinez-Perez ME, et al. Diagnosis of plus disease in retinopathy of prematurity using Retinal Image multiScale Analysis. Invest Ophth Vis Sci. 2005;46(12):4734–856.

53. Thyparampil PJ, Park Y, Martinez-Perez ME, et al. Plus disease in retinopathy of prematurity: quantitative analysis of vascular change. Am J Ophthalmol. 2010;150(4):468–75.

54. Wallace DK. Computer-assisted quantification of vascular tortuosity in retinopathy of prematurity (an American Ophthalmological Society thesis). Trans Am Ophthalmol Soc. 2007;105:594–615.

55. Cabrera MT, Freedman SF, Kiely AE, Chiang MF, Wallace DK. Combining ROPtool measurements of vascular tortuosity and width to quantify plus disease in retinopathy of prematurity. JAAPOS. 2011;15 (1):40–4.

56. Ng J, Clay ST, Barman SA, et al. Maximum likelihood estimation of vessel parameters from scale space analysis. Image Vis Comput. 2010;28:55–63.

57. Wilson CM, Cocker KD, Moseley M, et al. Computerized analysis of retinal blood vessel width and tortuosity in eyes at risk for retinopathy of prematurity. IOVS. 2008;49:3577–85.

58. Wilson CM. Classification and automated detection of the retinal vessels of premature infants with and without retinopathy of prematurity. PhD Thesis 2009.

59. Shah DN, Wilson CM, Ying GS, et al. Comparison of expert graders to computer-assisted image analysis of the retina in retinopathy of prematurity. Brit J Ophthalmol. 2011;95(10):1442–5.

60. Chiang MF, Gelman R, Martinez-Perez ME, et al. Image analysis for ROP diagnosis. JAAPOS. 2009;13:438–45.

61. Wittenberg LA, Jonsson NJ, Chan RVP, Chiang MF. Computer-based image analysis for plus disease and

pre plus disease in ROP. J Pediatr Ophthalmol Strabismus. 2012;49:11–9.

62. Wilson C, Theodoru M Cocker KD, Fielder AR The temporal retinal vessel angle and infants born preterm. Brit J Ophthalmol 2006;90(6):702–4.

63. Wong K, Ng J, Ells A, Fielder AR, Wilson CM. The temporal and nasal retinal and arteriolar and venular angles in infants born preterm. Brit J Ophthalmol. 2011;95(12):1723–7.

64. Oloumi F, Rangayyan RM, Ells AL. Assessment of vessel tortuosity in retinal images of preterm infants. Conf Proc IEEE Eng Med Biol Soc. 2014;2014:5410–3.

65. Oloumi F, Rangayyan RM, Ells AL. Quantification of the changes in the openness of the major temporal arcade in retinal fundus images of preterm infants with plus disease. Invest Ophthalmol Vis Sci. 2014;55(10):6728–35.

66. Wilson CM, Wong K, Ng J et al. Digital image analysis in ROP: a comparison of vessel selection methods. JAAPOS. 2012;16(3):223–9.

67. Lofqvist C, Hansen-Pupp I, Anderson E, et al. Validation of a new ROP screening method monitoring longitudinal postnatal weight and insulin-like growth factor 1. Arch Ophthalmol. 2009;127(5):622–7.

68. Hellstrom A, Hard AL, Engstrom E, et al. Early weight gain predicts retinopathy in preterm infants: new simple, efficient approach to screening. Pediatrics. 2009;123(4):e638–45.

69. Wu C, Vanderveen DK, Hellstrom A, Lofquist C, Smith LE. Longitudinal postnatal weight measurements for the prediction of retinopathy of prematurity. Arch Ophthalmol. 2010;128(4):443–7.

70. Binenbaum G, Ying GS, Quinn G, et al. A clinical prediction model to stratify retinopathy of prematurity risk using postnatal weight gain. Pediatrics. 2011;127(3):607–14.

71. Ells A, Guernsey DL, Wallace K, Zheng B, Voncer M, Allen A, Ingram A, DaSilva O, Siebert L, Sheidow T, Beis J. Robitaille JM Severe retinopathy of prematurity associated with FZD4 mutations. Ophthalmic Genet. 2010;31(1):37–43.

72. Hiraoka M, Bernstein DM, Trese MT et al. Insertion and deletion mutations in the dinucleotide repeat region of the Norrie disease gene in patients with advanced retinopathy of prematurity. J Hum Genet. 2001;46:178–181.

73. Jeffries AL. Canadian paediatric society, fetus and newborn committee. Paediatr Child Health. 2010;15:670.

74. Sociedad Argentina de Pediatria. Recommendations for retinopathy screening in at-risk populations. Arch Argent Pediatr. 2008;106:71–6.

75. Gobierno de Chile. Guia Clinica: Retinopatia del Prematurio 2005. http://www.redsalud.gov.ck/archiveos/guiasges/RetinopatiaPrematuorRMayo10.pdf.

76. Manejo de la retinopatía del recién nacido prematuro lineamientos técnicos. Secretaria de Salud de Mexico, 2007.

77. Colombian Guidelines for screening and treatment of ROP. 2010. Guia De Practica Clinica Retinpatia de le Prematuridad.

78. Visser I, Singh R, Young M, Lewis H. McKerrow N (ROP Working Group, South Africa). S Afr Med J. 2013;103:116–25.

Optical Coherence Tomography and Wide-Field Fluorescein Angiography in Retinopathy of Prematurity

4

Adam L. Rothman, Ramiro S. Maldonado, Lejla Vajzovic and Cynthia A. Toth

Abstract

The advent and adaptation of many imaging modalities promise to revolutionize our understanding of retinopathy of prematurity (ROP) by improving the detection, diagnosis, and monitoring of response to treatment of this disease. Diagnosis and classification of ROP traditionally relies on an eye exam by an ophthalmologist expert in this area who characterizes extent and character of retinal vascularization via indirect ophthalmoscopy. Many tools now exist that allow for data acquisition by nurses, technicians, and other trained staff with the images analyzed in a more centralized location. We will focus on two rapidly evolving technologies, optical coherence tomography (OCT), and wide field fluorescein angiography (FA), to better understand how these tools may change our current understanding and management of ROP.

Keywords

OCT—optical coherence tomography · Angiography · Retinopathy of prematurity (ROP) · Preterm · Wide-field

A.L. Rothman (✉) · R.S. Maldonado · L. Vajzovic
Ophthalmology, Duke University, 2301 Erwin Rd,
Durham, NC 27710, USA
e-mail: adam.rothman@duke.edu

R.S. Maldonado
e-mail: ramiro.maldonado@dm.duke.edu

L. Vajzovic
e-mail: lejla.vajzovic@dm.duke.edu

C.A. Toth
Ophthalmology and Biomedical Engineering,
Duke University, 2301 Erwin Rd, Durham,
NC 27710, USA
e-mail: cynthia.toth@dm.duke.edu

Optical Coherence Tomography

What Is Optical Coherence Tomography?

Optical coherence tomography (OCT) offers noninvasive, real-time, cross-sectional imaging of live tissue. It relies on interference patterns between light reflected from eye tissue compared to that reflected from a reference arm to obtain images with a resolution of a few microns [1]. First described by Huang et al. in 1991, the utility of

© Springer International Publishing AG 2017
Andrés Kychenthal B. and Paola Dorta S. (eds.), *Retinopathy of Prematurity*,
DOI 10.1007/978-3-319-52190-9_4

OCT in the field of ophthalmology was quickly realized when Swanson et al. provided the first high resolution, cross-sectional in vivo imaging of the human retina just 2 years later [2, 3]. Pathologies such as epiretinal membrane (ERM), macular holes, macular edema, and choroidal neovascularization can be imaged longitudinally to monitor disease progression [4–6]. These images can be processed and analyzed to further quantify the different compartments of the eye and, more specifically, layers of the retina [7]. Spectral domain (SD) OCT provides higher speed imaging and improved image quality, and the capability to sum serial frames to provide three-dimensional representations of the imaged material [8, 9]. Fully automated algorithms can be applied to segment, or outline, the individual retinal layers in both healthy and diseased eyes and sum serial frames to provide three-dimensional representations of the imaged material [10]. The promise of this imaging modality has led to many different commercial platforms, and conversion factors exist to reconcile quantitative measurements between the different devices [11].

Adapting Optical Coherence Tomography from Adult to Infant

Management of pathologies unique to the pediatric population demands the need to adapt OCT to children and infants. At first, only school age children were imaged with OCT as they could cooperate with the chin-rest apparatus designed for adults. Hess et al. first used a Carl Zeiss Meditec OCT system to image children ages 3–17 years old and identify a difference in macular and retinal nerve fiber layer (RNFL) thickness in children with and without glaucoma [12]. The relative ease of imaging school age children led to a normative database of macular thickness, RNFL thickness, and optic nerve topography in children aged 3–17 which demonstrated variation by race, axial length, and age in healthy children [13]. However, OCT imaging of infants presents unique challenges.

New hardware was required to obtain OCT images as traditional imaging apparatuses are vertically oriented and nonanesthetized and uncooperative infants must be imaged supine. In addition, rapid image acquisition is required due to the difficulty of movement in children [14]. At first, an unmounted Stratus tabletop system was utilized for infants under general anesthesia in the operating room [15]. Vinekar et al. disassembled the vertical camera unit of a Spectralis device and directed the freed camera on the nonanesthetized infant eye [16, 17]. More sophisticated devices have since been developed to image the infant eye. A portable, hand-held OCT (HHOCT) Bioptigen (Morrisville, NC, USA) system first used in infants by Maldonado et al. is now commonly accepted in the research community as the optimal OCT platform to image supine infants in various clinical and research scenarios. A movable imaging hand piece can be easily manipulated to an appropriate angle to align over a supine infant's eye and is connected via a flexible fiberoptic cable to a cart equipped with the SDOCT system and viewing screen. This mobile unit allows easy transportation between the clinic, operating room, and intensive care nursery for easy, noncontact, nonanesthetized supine imaging of infants [18, 19].

In addition to adapting the hardware to the infant population, the optics of the imaging system must also be modified to account for age-specific differences in axial length, refraction, and corneal curvature [20]. Hittner et al. first noted correlations between anterior chamber depth, keratometry readings and a history of ROP in 1979 [21]. Gordon and Donzis further characterized normal eye development in neonates by measuring an increase in axial length, decrease in corneal curvature, and subsequent hyperopic refractive shift [22]. Further studies have demonstrated that vitreous chamber length in preterm infants increased most rapidly from 30 to 55 weeks post-menstrual age (PMA) [23]. Because of these unique properties, optical formulae derived from Gullstrand's model eye, which employs estimates to image the infant retina with a summary simplified lens, are employed by the premature-eye model developed by Maldonado et al. [20, 24]. These estimates may slightly vary in the ROP population. Although corneal curvature is normally the most significant contributor to changes in refraction in the neonatal population, keratometry is not related to ROP stages; however, at and after term, axial length changes may vary proportional to severity of ROP [25]. Now, based on the aforementioned optical systems, an age-specific method to image premature infants, newborns, and infants has been developed [20].

Developmental Retinal and Optic Nerve Microanatomy Observed on Optical Coherence Tomography in Preterm Infants

To better understand the structural and functional changes associated with ROP, one must first understand the normal microanatomy of the retina and its growth at an early age. Portable HHOCT systems have allowed for imaging of preterm and full term infants during the dynamic neonatal period. In particular, multiple studies both comparing the microanatomy of preterm infants with their full term counterparts as well as monitoring changes in microanatomy of preterm infants over time have increased our knowledge of normal retinal development [26–28]. Only by understanding normal retinal development can we detect, diagnosis, and monitor the changes caused by ROP.

The fovea undergoes extensive maturation changes during the neonatal period. Hendrickson and Yuodelis first described human foveal development in cadaver eyes and noted thick ganglion cells and the absence of rods at the site that becomes the recognizable fovea by 22 weeks PMA [29]. Rather than studying human cadavers, OCT imaging of preterm infants reveals the changes in retinal microanatomy that typically occur in utero. Maldonado et al. reported the first in vivo tracking of foveal development by monitoring the displacement of inner retinal layers and appearance of a thin photoreceptor layer in preterm infants imaged with OCT. Three-dimensional mapping revealed centrifugal migration of the inner retinal layers over time from the fovea with concurrent centripetal formation of the inner segment/outer segment band [28].

Immunohistologic evaluation of postmortem infant retinas further reveals the intricate formation and movement of the various components of the retinal layers in the macula [30]. Vajzovic et al. have validated the use of OCT to monitor these changes by correlating histologic findings with OCT images [27]. On OCT and matching histology, they found deepening of the foveal pit due to displacement of inner retinal layers in preterm infants with concurrent growth of the photoreceptor outer segments separating the photoreceptor inner segments from the retinal pigment epithelium (Fig. 4.1). Vajzovic has also demonstrated delayed photoreceptor maturation in preterm infants when compared to term infants of the same age (at 37–42 weeks PMA) doi: 10.1167/iovs.14-16021. Others have also documented the maturation of the photoreceptors through OCT imaging over the first 17 postnatal months [31].

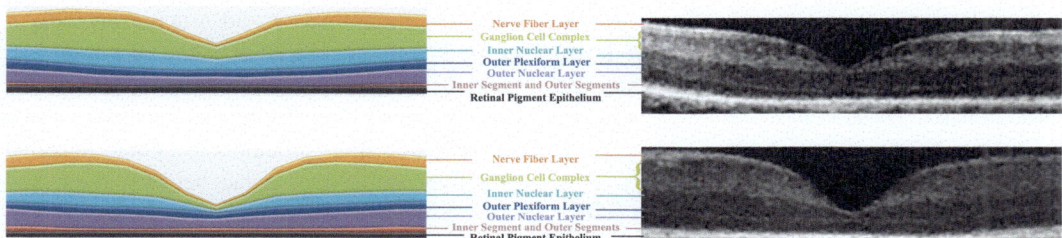

Fig. 4.1 *Top*, Color illustration of retina maturation at 33–36 weeks post-menstrual age (PMA) with sample spectral-domain optical coherence tomography (SDOCT) cross-sectional B-scan of a former 1640 g, 30 week PMA gestational age infant imaged at 33 weeks PMA with no retinopathy of prematurity (ROP). Note the shallow foveal pit, persistence of inner retinal layers, and lack of inner segment band at the center of the fovea. *Bottom*, Color illustration of retina maturation at 40–42 weeks PMA with sample SDOCT B-scan of a former 880 g, 28 week PMA gestational age infant with stage 2, pre-plus ROP imaged at 41 weeks PMA. The foveal pit has greater depth and there is inner retinal layers displacement from the foveal center when compared to top B-scan

Recent advances in enhanced depth imaging OCT have allowed for better visualization of the choroid-scleral junction and an appreciation for the development of the macula's vascular supply [32]. Moreno et al. measured significantly thinner choroid in young preterm infants (less than 37 weeks PMA) versus term-aged preterm infants (37–42 weeks PMA), term infants, and adult subjects. In addition, they found term-aged preterm infants had thinner choroid than term infants [26]. Choroid thickness then continues to increase from early childhood through adolescence [33].

Changes in neurosensory tissue of the retina over time can also be appreciated with SDOCT. Samarawickrama et al. measured larger cup-to-disc ratios on OCT in children with a history of low birth weight, short birth length, and a small head circumference [34]. However, analysis of color fundus photography of full term infants did not reveal any differences in optic disc measurements by sex or birth weight [35]. Additionally, RNFL is thinner in school-aged children who were born preterm which correlates with foveal thickness and visual acuity [36]. Optical coherence tomography has also identified differences in optic nerve head parameters by race [37]. Recently, Tong et al. found a larger cup and cup-to-disc ratio in preterm infants imaged with HHOCT compared to fullterm infants as well as a correlation between preterm optic cup-to-disc ratio and cognitive development at 18–24 months PMA [38]. Recently, these differences in RNFL thickness between term and preterm infants have been measured while still in the nursery, with thinner RNFL relating to both brain structure and neurodevelopment doi: 10.1016/j.ajo.2015.01.017 and 10.1016/j.ajo.2015.09.015.

Optical Coherence Tomography in ROP

Because there is such a strong correlation between structure and functional outcomes in patients with ROP, OCT promises to revolutionize the treatment of ROP by providing valuable subclinical information about eye morphology [39, 40]. Joshi et al. used time domain OCT to confirm absence of macular involvement of stage 4A retinal detachments before repair by pars plana vitrectomy and first suggested that subclinical anatomic abnormalities that can be observed by OCT may explain differences in outcomes for stage 4A vitrectomies [15]. Chavala et al. further demonstrated the utility of SDOCT as an adjunct to traditional examination techniques. They identified retinoschisis and preretinal structures believed to represent preretinal fibrovascular proliferation that were not identified by conventional examination in three patients with advanced ROP (Fig. 4.2, top left) [41]. Muni et al. similarly report a case series where ROP progressed after laser photocoagulation presumably due to tractional retinoschisis observed by OCT that remained undetected by indirect ophthalmoscopy [42].

A more thorough study by Lee et al. evaluated 76 eyes of 38 infants by both HHOCT and traditional indirect ophthalmoscopy during routine ROP exams. Masked graders then qualitatively graded the OCT scans for the presence of preretinal and retina findings. They found that 39% of examinations revealed intraretinal cystoid structures and 32% had an ERM on OCT while these features were never identified by conventional exam. However, indirect ophthalmoscopy was able to identify ROP stage and status of plus disease while OCT did not reveal this clinical information [43].

Vinekar et al. similarly compared the SDOCT imaging of patients with ROP to traditional indirect ophthalmoscopy. They identified and described intraretinal cystoid structures in 29% of subjects with stage 2 ROP, none of whom had cystoid macular edema (CME) identified on clinical exam. They further characterized these intraretinal cystoid structures as either elongated with hyper-reflective septae between them and causing foveal deformation and bulging (Fig. 4.2, top right) or fewer intraretinal cystoid structures which did not cause foveal deformation. Additionally, they note that no eyes with stage 1 ROP or without ROP had these findings [16].

Maldonado et al. further characterized this CME in preterm infants. They found CME in 50% of the 42 preterm infants included in their study

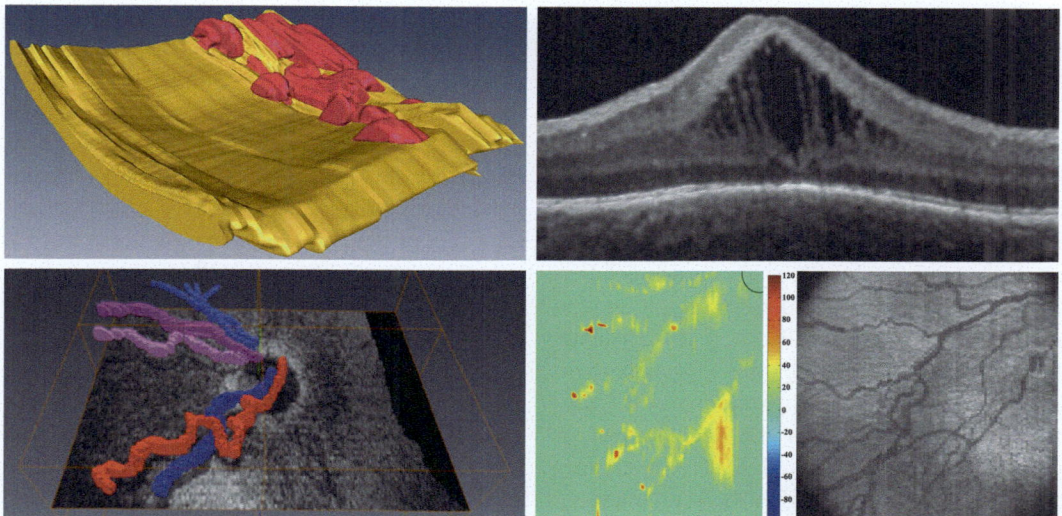

Fig. 4.2 *Top left*, Three-dimensional representation of clinically undetected preretinal structures identified using spectral-domain optical coherence tomography (SDOCT) in a former 650 g, 23 week post-menstrual age (PMA) gestational age infant imaged at 37 weeks PMA after receiving laser treatment for aggressive posterior retinopathy of prematurity (ROP). *Top right*, SDOCT B-scan reveals cross section of a former 940 g, 27 week PMA gestational age imaged at 46 weeks PMA demonstrating severe cystoid macular edema. Note the elongated hypo-reflective spaces with intermittent hyper-reflective stranding within the inner nuclear layer. *Bottom left*, Three-dimensional representation of retinal vessels created from SDOCT scan of a former 700 g, 25 week PMA gestational age infant imaged at 42 week PMA with plus disease. Tortuosity can be appreciated in all dimensions, as opposed to traditional *en face* examination. *Bottom right*, retinal surface map of a former 478 g, 23 week PMA gestational age infant imaged at 34 weeks PMA with plus disease represents vessel elevation, as a consequence of vessel dilation, from the inner surface of the retina. Image was produced by segmentation of SDOCT scan and corresponds with adjacent *en face* vascular pattern

which most commonly appeared as multiple elongated cystoid structures within the inner nuclear layer (INL). The presence of CME was not associated with ROP outcomes; however, central foveal thickness, the thickness of the INL, and the foveal-to-parafoveal ratio all served as markers of CME severity. While these measures were greater in eyes that required laser photocoagulation or developed plus disease or stage 3 ROP, there was wide overlap of measurements between ROP severities. However, there were no associations between CME and any systemic parameters [44].

The etiology of subclinical CME in subjects with ROP remains unexplained. Some hypothesize that a higher concentration of vascular endothelial growth factor (VEGF) increases vascular permeability and the subsequent formation of cystoid structures. Maldonado et al. posit the CME "may also reflect the contribution of increased intracapillary hydrostatic pressure as a result [of] vascular congestion from plus disease" [44]. In another report, one infant developed CME after bevacizumab treatment (used off-label as anti-VEGF therapy for ROP) while three infants did not experience CME resolution after bevacizumab therapy. Another possibility is these cystoid structures form secondary to mechanical traction exerted on the retina [16]. Although there are no recognized markers of systemic health associated with CME, a case report of an infant with hemochromatosis and severe, bilateral CME that resolved with liver transplant suggests there may be other unidentified systemic health factors associated with CME [45]. It appears that CME does resolve on its own; however, the long term clinical implications remain unknown and require further study [16, 44, 46] doi: 10.1016/j.ophtha.2014.09.022 and 10.1097/IAE. 0000000000000579.

OCT has increased our understanding of abnormal development of multiple tissue layers of the infant retina that can be affected by premature birth or by ROP. The most prominent retinal finding on OCT in children with a history of preterm birth and ROP is the notable persistence of inner retinal layers. Recchia et al, in older children and adults, reported an abnormal foveal contour and the persistence of inner retinal layers in those with a history of ROP [47]. Optical coherence tomography allows for an appreciation for the shallower and wider foveal pit in this population [48]. Additionally, there is persistence of inner retinal layers regardless of maximum ROP stage observed [46]. Retinopathy of prematurity appears to affect the development of neurosensory tissue as well. There is thinner RNFL in school-aged children born prematurely with stage 3 and 4 ROP [49]. Tong et al. measured a shallower cup depth in stage 3 ROP or ROP requiring treatment using OCT [38]. Last, while Wu et al. noted a thinner choroid in patients who had undergone treatment for ROP as well as an inverse relationship between choroid thickness and best corrected visual acuity, Park et al. only noted a trend in thinner temporal choroid for children with worsening ROP stage [50, 51].

Evaluation of vasculature is critical to the diagnosis and management of ROP. To date, OCT has only served as a useful adjunct to the gold standard of indirect ophthalmoscopy when characterizing the vasculature and evaluating treatment options [52]. One limitation of this technology has been the inability to reliably characterize ROP stage and determine the status of plus disease. Maldonado et al. recently created a Vascular Abnormality Score on OCT (VASO) in order to quantify vascular and perivascular OCT findings associated with ROP. In contrast to *en face* color fundus photography or indirect ophthalmoscopy, OCT appreciates three-dimensional vessel distortion, including in the anterior–posterior direction (Fig. 4.2, bottom left). This VASO tool is useful to qualitatively evaluate OCT scans for vessel elevation and severity of elevation, scalloping of the inner plexiform layer and outer plexiform layer, hypo-reflective vessels, and perivascular spaces. Patients with plus disease had a significantly higher VASO due to a greater incidence of vessel

elevation, hypo-reflective vessels, and scalloped retinal layers. In addition, retinal surface maps of subjects with plus disease demonstrated greater surface elevation (Fig. 4.2, bottom right). While the VASO system and retinal surface maps require further validation before being incorporated into clinical practice, these tools suggest OCT can provide new information regarding the vascular abnormalities of ROP [53].

Optical coherence tomography has rapidly evolved over the past 20 years and its clinical applications will likely expand in the future. While the initial cost of equipment may limit some health care systems from implementing this technology, the availability of OCT continues to spread. Intraoperative OCT can assist in the management of the complications of ROP, such as retinal detachment and ERMs [41, 54]. OCT was first introduced in the operating room with the same portable, hand-held system brought to the nursery to image infants and children undergoing exams under anesthesia [55]. It has now been integrated into the surgical microscope to allow live cross-sectional imaging while operating [56–58]. Color Doppler OCT, first described in 1997, images fluid flow which allows for in vivo imaging of blood flow and subsequent three-dimension reconstruction of blood vessels [59–61]. While Doppler OCT has not yet been investigated in the context of ROP, one can easily appreciate the utility of cross-sectional visualization of blood flow in this population. In addition, advances to the actual OCT apparatus such as the development of a hand-held swept source OCT system will allow for faster data acquisition with greater precision [62]. With so many advances on the horizon, OCT promises to revolutionize the diagnosis and management of ROP.

Wide Field Imaging and Fluorescein Angiography

What Is Wide Field Imaging?

Evaluation of the peripheral retina is important when diagnosing and monitoring treatment for patients with many pathologies, including ROP. When discussing the field of view obtained by an imaging device, one refers to the external angle of light as it enters the eye, which is determined by the focal length, dimensions of the imaged object, and lens power. Fundus imaging has traditionally been limited to approximately 30° field of view [63]. Fields of view have expanded as individuals have altered the optic systems of devices. For example, Pomerantzeff could image nearly 150° of the retina with his contact lens-based system that relied on both trans-pupillary and trans-scleral illumination [64].

The most commonly accepted wide-field imaging tool currently in practice for the ROP population is the RetCam 120 (Clarity Medical Systems, Inc., Pleasanton, CA) which obtains up to 130° digital fundus photographs with the assistance of different contact lenses. First commercially available in 1997, RetCam was quickly adopted by the pediatric community as it allows portable, supine imaging of the peripheral retina. Because the image quality depends on having a clear lens, RetCam typically produces much poorer images in the adult population [63]. The newer nonmydriatic Optomap Panoramic 200 scanning laser ophthalmoscope (Optos P200, Optos, Dumferline, Scotland, United Kingdom) allows for 180°–200° fundus imaging and is less susceptible than fundus photo to media opacities such as cataract [65]. The Optos's ellipsoid mirror creates two focal points which allows for greater fields of view [63].

Several advantages and disadvantages exist when comparing the feasibility of the RetCam and Optos P200 MA to image infants. The Optos P200 MA allows for greater field of view while the RetCam will have more difficulty imaging multiple areas simultaneously. As RetCam relies on incandescent light while Optos uses dual laser illumination with a more uniform focus, RetCam may have a more difficult time imaging infants with media opacities or small pupils. Image acquisition time, very important when imaging noncooperative infants with eye movement, is longer for the RetCam system as the user must refocus and reapply coupling media. However,

the RetCam system is portable which allows easy imaging of supine infants in unique settings, such as the nursery; the Optos system is traditionally limited to outpatient imaging and requires infants to be held in an upright position. The noncontact image acquisition of Optos may reduce the drawback of changes in vessel appearance from ocular compression but also may introduce artifacts if there is matter between the device and eye [66]. Because there are two laser wavelengths used with Optos, this imaging system does not accurately portray colors.

Wide Field Imaging and ROP Telemedicine

The growing field of telemedicine has benefited from these digital wide-field imaging tools. These devices obtain fundus photographs and videos of patients so they may be analyzed off-site. While these technologies can be performed by a technician or nurse with a more flexible schedule than a pediatric ophthalmologist, the initial cost of the equipment can be expensive and they offer less complete visualization of the fundus and subsequently documentation of ROP compared to the gold standard of indirect ophthalmoscopy [67]. By comparing off-site digital photograph reading to traditional indirect ophthalmoscopy and determining the sensitivity and specificity in detecting ROP, we can decide if digital wide-field imaging can serve as a screening tool for ROP.

Multiple studies have demonstrated variable sensitivity and specificity of ROP diagnoses by RetCam versus indirect ophthalmoscopy [68–71]. Discrepancies in study protocols and aims when comparing published results, such as sensitivity and specificity of ROP diagnoses by RetCam, has led to a standardized, prospective, multicenter trial entitled "Telemedicine Approaches to Evaluating Acute-phase ROP (e-ROP, www.clinicaltrials. gov identifier NCT01264276)." The trial will "evaluate the validity, reliability, feasibility, safety, and relative cost-effectiveness of a retinopathy of prematurity (ROP) telemedicine evaluation system to detect eyes of at-risk babies who meet referral warranted ROP (RW-ROP) criteria and therefore need a diagnostic evaluation by an ophthalmologist experienced in ROP." With a planned enrollment of 2500 preterm infants independently examined via indirect ophthalmoscopy and by RetCam digital images at a remote location, this study should determine whether digital wide-field imaging can effectively serve as a surrogate for traditional on-site ophthalmologic examination.

Wide-Field Fluorescein Angiography and ROP

The incorporation of FA into wide-field imaging promises to change how we monitor treatment of ROP. In 2006, Ng et al. first presented the feasibility of imaging the peripheral vasculature by applying the fluorescein angiographic RetCam digital system [72]. Lepore et al. have since provided a more thorough atlas of the vascular abnormalities associated with severe ROP. They obtained images before and after laser photocoagulation and believe this helped determine the efficacy of the ablation. Wide variability in the time lapse from intravenous injection to the arteriolar phase and then venular phase suggests great variability in blood flow with these infants, including in the choroid. The authors note irregular branching patterns at the vascular–avascular junction and even more variable vascular findings, including dilatation of capillaries, capillary tuft formation, and rosary-bead-like hyperfluorescent lesions in the vascular retina and posterior pole [73]. Purcaro et al. provide an additional case series demonstrating the efficacy of RetCam FA to characterize vessel branching at the vascular–avascular junction and suggest dye leakage may be a sign of progression to severe ROP [74]. Additionally, RetCam FA can identify vascular changes before they are detected with traditional indirect ophthalmoscopy [75].

Several case series suggest wide-field FA is a useful perioperative tool when monitoring the treatment for different sequelae of ROP. For example, Yokoi et al. obtained RetCam 120 FA images before and after laser and surgical treatment for six eyes with aggressive posterior ROP. Pre-operatively, they could appreciate capillary nonperfusion, shunting in vascularized retina, and a circumferential demarcation line while after treatment they could appreciate a capillary-free zone, poorly developed disorganized vessels, and an inhomogeneous capillary bed [76]. The same research group reports the utility of RetCam120 FA when securing sclera buckles due to stage 4A ROP. All five eyes that underwent scleral buckling demonstrated pre-operative fluorescein leakage from fibrovascular tissue. Between 7 and 20 days after successful surgery, four eyes had decreased leakage while one eye had no leakage [77].

The introduction of bevacizumab as an off-label treatment for ROP offers another opportunity to advance patient care with the assistance of wide-field FA. Wide-field FA can successfully confirm the absence of pathologic neovascularization and document vascular density and evolution of anomalous vascular patterns after bevacizumab treatment [78]. However, additional studies suggest that wide-field FA can help monitor for disease progression that may occur after treatment because of the potential for transient blockage of VEGF with bevacizumab versus the long-acting down-regulation associated with laser photocoagulation (Fig. 4.3). Hoang et al. provide a case report of circumferential anastomosis at the bevacizumab-induced regression site with future anterior involvement observed by RetCam FA. They report an infant with zone II, stage 3 plus disease responded well to intravitreous bevacizumab. However, 2 months after treatment, a second stage 3 complex formed anterior to the original lesion with RetCam FA demonstrating "anterior extraretinal fibrovascular proliferation with leakage and a more posterior circumferential vascular ring with associated telangiectasis but without leakage" [79]. Hu et al. have additionally documented this late reactivation of disease after transient regression following bevacizumab as observed with RetCam FA [80]. Visualization of peripheral retina hemodynamics with the assistance of wide-field FA clearly serves as a clinically relevant adjunct to traditional indirect ophthalmoscopy.

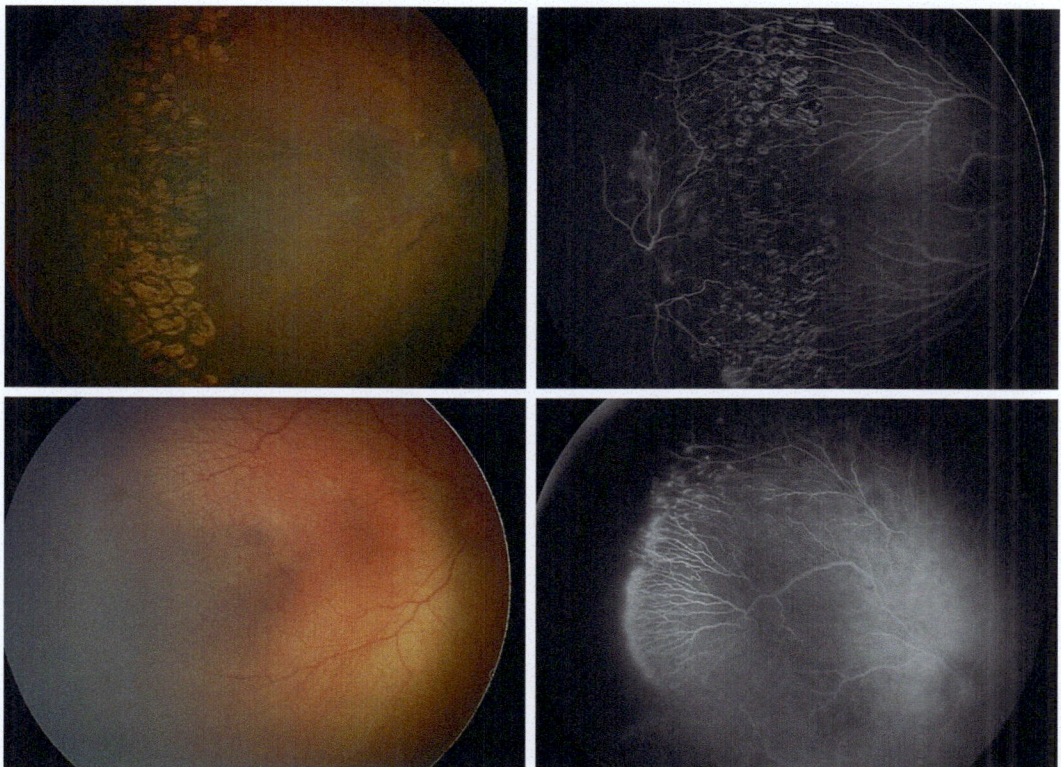

Fig. 4.3 *Top* panels show fundus and fluorescein angiography photographs of the right eye of an infant after conventional laser and intravitreal bevacizumab therapy for stage 3 zone 2 ROP. The infant was born at 25 weeks' gestational age, with a birth weight of 570 g. These follow-up photographs show areas of peripheral retinal laser photocoagulation and interestingly neovascularization anterior to laser treated area. *Bottom* panels show fundus and fluorescein angiography photographs of the right eye of an infant with history of intravitreal bevacizumab therapy for stage 3 zone 1 ROP. The infant was born at 26 weeks' gestational age, with a birth weight of 850 g. Although intravitreal bevacizumab treatment was initially effective in inducing regression of ROP, the effect was transient. Recurrent neovascularization (*bottom right*), which was noted at 48 weeks PMA, is far more visible on the angiogram than on the color fundus photograph (*bottom left*)

Adapting the ultra-wide field Optos system to incorporate FA can further visualize peripheral retinal vasculature. Manivannan et al. first report the use of ultra-wide field fluorescein angiography in 2005 by imaging patients with diabetic retinopathy and uveitis with the Optos Panoramic 200. The increased field of view allowed for evaluation of peripheral retinal nonperfusion as well as simultaneous comparisons of distant lesions [81]. Recently, Fung et al. report the successful FA imaging of three infants with ROP with the Optos ultra-wide field view SLO. They believe that such great visualization of neovascularization in their case study allows for accurate identification of avascular versus vascular retina for targeted laser treatment. Additionally, intravenous access was not required as oral fluorescein was mixed with infant formula milk [82].

Conclusion

Recent advances in imaging promise to change the diagnosis, treatment, and monitoring of ROP. OCT allows for in vivo cross-sectional retinal imaging of infants in the nursery and a better understanding of how ROP can disrupt normal development of retinal and macular microanatomy; vascular abnormalities can be reconstructed in three-dimensions and appreciated from other perspectives than in the traditional *en face* viewing. Wide-field OCT imaging in the ROP population may allow cross-sectional visualization peripheral neovascular tissue. The digitalization of imaging allows for off-site acquisition of large field-of-view fundus images which can then be analyzed remotely. These wide-field imaging tools can then be paired with FA to monitor vascular flow, abnormal vascular patterns, avascular retina, neovascularization, and leakage. The transition of OCT and wide-field FA from research to clinical practice will serve as an indispensable adjunct to traditional imaging methods for infants with ROP.

References

1. Fujimoto JG. Optical coherence tomography for ultrahigh resolution in vivo imaging. Nat Biotechnol. 2003;21:1361–7.
2. Huang D, Swanson EA, Lin CP, et al. Optical coherence tomography. Science (New York, NY). 1991;254:1178–81.
3. Swanson EA, Izatt JA, Hee MR, et al. In vivo retinal imaging by optical coherence tomography. Opt Lett. 1993;18:1864–6.
4. Puliafito CA, Hee MR, Lin CP, et al. Imaging of macular diseases with optical coherence tomography. Ophthalmology. 1995;102:217–29.
5. Hee MR, Puliafito CA, Wong C, et al. Quantitative assessment of macular edema with optical coherence tomography. Arch Ophthalmol. 1995;113:1019–29.
6. Daniel E, Toth CA, Grunwald JE, et al. Risk of scar in the comparison of age-related macular degeneration treatments trials. Ophthalmology. 2014;121:656–66.
7. Schuman JS, Hee MR, Puliafito CA, et al. Quantification of nerve fiber layer thickness in normal and glaucomatous eyes using optical coherence tomography. Arch Ophthalmol. 1995;113:586–96.
8. Fercher AF, Hitzenberger CK, Kamp G, El-Zaiat SY. Measurement of intraocular distances by backscattering spectral interferometry. Optics Communications. 1995;117:43–8.
9. de Boer JF, Cense B, Park BH, Pierce MC, Tearney GJ, Bouma BE. Improved signal-to-noise ratio in spectral-domain compared with time-domain optical coherence tomography. Opt Lett. 2003;28:2067–9.
10. Lee JY, Chiu SJ, Srinivasan PP, et al. Fully automatic software for retinal thickness in eyes with diabetic macular edema from images acquired by cirrus and spectralis systems. Invest Ophthalmol Vis Sci. 2013;54:7595–602.
11. Folgar FA, Yuan EL, Farsiu S, Toth CA. Lateral and axial measurement differences between spectral-domain optical coherence tomography systems. J Biomed Opt. 2014;19:16014.
12. Hess DB, Asrani SG, Bhide MG, Enyedi LB, Stinnett SS, Freedman SF. Macular and retinal nerve fiber layer analysis of normal and glaucomatous eyes in children using optical coherence tomography. Am J Ophthalmol. 2005;139:509–17.
13. El-Dairi MA, Asrani SG, Enyedi LB, Freedman SF. Optical coherence tomography in the eyes of normal children. Arch Ophthalmol. 2009;127:50–8.
14. Chong GT, Farsiu S, Freedman SF, et al. Abnormal foveal morphology in ocular albinism imaged with spectral-domain optical coherence tomography. Arch Ophthalmol. 2009;127:37–44.
15. Joshi MM, Trese MT, Capone A Jr. Optical coherence tomography findings in stage 4A retinopathy of prematurity: a theory for visual variability. Ophthalmology. 2006;113:657–60.
16. Vinekar A, Avadhani K, Sivakumar M, et al. Understanding clinically undetected macular changes in early retinopathy of prematurity on spectral domain optical coherence tomography. Invest Ophthalmol Vis Sci. 2011;52:5183–8.
17. Vinekar A, Sivakumar M, Shetty R, et al. A novel technique using spectral-domain optical coherence tomography (Spectralis, SD-OCT + HRA) to image supine non-anaesthetized infants: utility demonstrated in aggressive posterior retinopathy of prematurity. Eye (London, England). 2010;24:379–82.
18. Scott AW, Farsiu S, Enyedi LB, Wallace DK, Toth CA. Imaging the infant retina with a hand-held spectral-domain optical coherence tomography device. Am J Ophthalmol. 2009;147(364–73):e2.
19. Rothman AL, Folgar FA, Tong AY, Toth CA. Spectral domain optical coherence tomography characterization of pediatric epiretinal membranes. Retina (Philadelphia, Pa) 2014.
20. Maldonado RS, Izatt JA, Sarin N, et al. Optimizing hand-held spectral domain optical coherence tomography imaging for neonates, infants, and children. Invest Ophthalmol Vis Sci. 2010;51:2678–85.
21. Hittner HM, Rhodes LM, McPherson AR. Anterior segment abnormalities in cicatricial retinopathy of prematurity. Ophthalmology. 1979;86:803–16.
22. Gordon RA, Donzis PB. Refractive development of the human eye. Arch Ophthalmol. 1985;103:785–9.
23. Mactier H, Maroo S, Bradnam M, Hamilton R. Ocular biometry in preterm infants: implications for estimation of retinal illuminance. Invest Ophthalmol Vis Sci. 2008;49:453–7.
24. Gullstrand A. Appendices II and IV. In: Southall JPC, editor. Helmholtz's treatise on physiological optics. Menasha, WI: Optical Society of America; 1909.

25. Cook A, White S, Batterbury M, Clark D. Ocular growth and refractive error development in premature infants with or without retinopathy of prematurity. Invest Ophthalmol Vis Sci. 2008;49:5199–207.

26. Moreno TA, O'Connell RV, Chiu SJ, et al. Choroid development and feasibility of choroidal imaging in the preterm and term infants utilizing SD-OCT. Invest Ophthalmol Vis Sci. 2013;54:4140–7.

27. Vajzovic L, Hendrickson AE, O'Connell RV, et al. Maturation of the human fovea: correlation of spectral-domain optical coherence tomography findings with histology. Am J Ophthalmol. 2012;154 (779–89):e2.

28. Maldonado RS, O'Connell RV, Sarin N, et al. Dynamics of human foveal development after premature birth. Ophthalmology. 2011;118:2315–25.

29. Hendrickson AE, Yuodelis C. The morphological development of the human fovea. Ophthalmology. 1984;91:603–12.

30. Hendrickson A, Possin D, Vajzovic L, Toth CA. Histologic development of the human fovea from midgestation to maturity. Am J Ophthalmol. 2012;154(767–78):e2.

31. Dubis AM, Costakos DM, Subramaniam CD, et al. Evaluation of normal human foveal development using optical coherence tomography and histologic examination. Arch Ophthalmol. 2012;130:1291–300.

32. Yiu G, Pecen P, Sarin N, et al. Characterization of the choroid-scleral junction and suprachoroidal layer in healthy individuals on enhanced-depth imaging optical coherence tomography. JAMA Ophthalmol. 2013.

33. Read SA, Collins MJ, Vincent SJ, Alonso-Caneiro D. Choroidal thickness in childhood. Invest Ophthalmol Vis Sci. 2013;54:3586–93.

34. Samarawickrama C, Huynh SC, Liew G, Burlutsky G, Mitchell P. Birth weight and optic nerve head parameters. Ophthalmology. 2009;116:1112–8.

35. Kandasamy Y, Smith R, Wright IM, Hartley L. Optic disc measurements in full term infants. Br J Ophthalmol. 2012;96:662–4.

36. Wang J, Spencer R, Leffler JN, Birch EE. Characteristics of peripapillary retinal nerve fiber layer in preterm children. Am J Ophthalmol. 2012;153(850–5):e1.

37. Allingham MJ, Cabrera MT, O'Connell RV, et al. Racial variation in optic nerve head parameters quantified in healthy newborns by handheld spectral domain optical coherence tomography. Journal of AAPOS: Off publ Am Assoc Pediatr Ophthalmol Strabismus/Am Assoc Pediatr Ophthalmol Strabismus. 2013;17:501–6.

38. Tong AY, El-Dairi M, Maldonado RS, et al. Evaluation of optic nerve development in preterm and term infants using handheld spectral-domain optical coherence tomography. Ophthalmology. 2014.

39. Maldonado RS, Toth CA. Optical coherence tomography in retinopathy of prematurity: looking beyond the vessels. Clin Perinatol. 2013;40:271–96.

40. Wallace DK, Bremer DL, Good WV, et al. Correlation of recognition visual acuity with posterior retinal structure in advanced retinopathy of prematurity. Arch Ophthalmol. 2012;130:1512–6.

41. Chavala SH, Farsiu S, Maldonado R, Wallace DK, Freedman SF, Toth CA. Insights into advanced retinopathy of prematurity using handheld spectral domain optical coherence tomography imaging. Ophthalmology. 2009;116:2448–56.

42. Muni RH, Kohly RP, Charonis AC, Lee TC. Retinoschisis detected with handheld spectral-domain optical coherence tomography in neonates with advanced retinopathy of prematurity. Arch Ophthalmol. 2010;128:57–62.

43. Lee AC, Maldonado RS, Sarin N, et al. Macular features from spectral-domain optical coherence tomography as an adjunct to indirect ophthalmoscopy in retinopathy of prematurity. Retina (Philadelphia, Pa). 2011;31:1470–82.

44. Maldonado RS, O'Connell R, Ascher SB, et al. Spectral-domain optical coherence tomographic assessment of severity of cystoid macular edema in retinopathy of prematurity. Arch Ophthalmol. 2012;130:569–78.

45. Maldonado RS, Freedman SF, Cotten CM, Ferranti JM, Toth CA. Reversible retinal edema in an infant with neonatal hemochromatosis and liver failure. J Am Assoc Pediatr Ophthalmol Strabismus. 2011;15:91–3.

46. Dubis AM, Subramaniam CD, Godara P, Carroll J, Costakos DM. Subclinical macular findings in infants screened for retinopathy of prematurity with spectral-domain optical coherence tomography. Ophthalmology. 2013;120:1665–71.

47. Recchia FM, Recchia CC. Foveal dysplasia evident by optical coherence tomography in patients with a history of retinopathy of prematurity. Retina (Philadelphia, Pa). 2007;27:1221–6.

48. Hammer DX, Iftimia NV, Ferguson RD, et al. Foveal fine structure in retinopathy of prematurity: an adaptive optics Fourier domain optical coherence tomography study. Invest Ophthalmol Vis Sci. 2008;49:2061–70.

49. Akerblom H, Holmstrom G, Eriksson U, Larsson E. Retinal nerve fibre layer thickness in school-aged prematurely-born children compared to children born at term. Br J Ophthalmol. 2012;96:956–60.

50. Park KA, Oh SY. Analysis of spectral-domain optical coherence tomography in preterm children: retinal layer thickness and choroidal thickness profiles. Invest Ophthalmol Vis Sci. 2012;53:7201–7.

51. Wu WC, Shih CP, Wang NK, et al. Choroidal thickness in patients with a history of retinopathy of prematurity. JAMA Ophthalmol. 2013;131:1451–3.

52. The international classification of retinopathy of prematurity revisited. Arch Ophthalmol. 2005;123:991–9

53. Maldonado RS, Yuan E, Tran-Viet D, et al. Three-dimensional assessment of vascular and

perivascular characteristics in subjects with retinopathy of prematurity. Ophthalmology. 2014.

54. Hahn P, Migacz J, O'Connell R, Maldonado RS, Izatt JA, Toth CA. The use of optical coherence tomography in intraoperative ophthalmic imaging. Ophthalmic surg Lasers Imaging: Off J Int Soc Imaging Eye. 2011;42(Suppl):S85–94.

55. Dayani PN, Maldonado R, Farsiu S, Toth CA. Intraoperative use of handheld spectral domain optical coherence tomography imaging in macular surgery. Retina (Philadelphia, Pa). 2009;29:1457–68.

56. Ehlers JP, Tao YK, Farsiu S, Maldonado R, Izatt JA, Toth CA. Integration of a spectral domain optical coherence tomography system into a surgical microscope for intraoperative imaging. Invest Ophthalmol Vis Sci. 2011;52:3153–9.

57. Hahn P, Migacz J, O'Connell R, Izatt JA, Toth CA. Unprocessed real-time imaging of vitreoretinal surgical maneuvers using a microscope-integrated spectral-domain optical coherence tomography system. Graefe's Arch Clin Exp Ophthalmol = Albrecht von Graefes Archiv fur klinische und experimentelle Ophthalmologie. 2013;251:213–20.

58. Hahn P, Migacz J, O'Donnell R, et al. Preclinical evaluation and intraoperative human retinal imaging with a high-resolution microscope-integrated spectral domain optical coherence tomography device. Retina (Philadelphia, Pa). 2013;33:1328–37.

59. Chen Z, Milner TE, Dave D, Nelson JS. Optical Doppler tomographic imaging of fluid flow velocity in highly scattering media. Opt Lett. 1997;22:64–6.

60. Izatt JA, Kulkarni MD, Yazdanfar S, Barton JK, Welch AJ. In vivo bidirectional color Doppler flow imaging of picoliter blood volumes using optical coherence tomography. Opt Lett. 1997;22:1439–41.

61. Kehlet Barton J, Izatt JA, Kulkarni MD, Yazdanfar S, Welch AJ. Three-dimensional reconstruction of blood vessels from in vivo color Doppler optical coherence tomography images. Dermatology (Basel, Switzerland). 1999;198:355–61.

62. Lu CD, Kraus MF, Potsaid B, et al. Handheld ultrahigh speed swept source optical coherence tomography instrument using a MEMS scanning mirror. Biomed Opt Express. 2013;5:293–311.

63. Witmer MT, Kiss S. Wide-field imaging of the retina. Surv Ophthalmol. 2013;58:143–54.

64. Pomerantzeff O. Equator-plus camera. Invest Ophthalmol. 1975;14:401–6.

65. Neubauer AS, Kernt M, Haritoglou C, Priglinger SG, Kampik A, Ulbig MW. Nonmydriatic screening for diabetic retinopathy by ultra-widefield scanning laser ophthalmoscopy (Optomap). Graefe's Arch Clin Exp Ophthalmol. 2008;246:229–35.

66. Fung TH, Yusuf IH, Smith LM, Brett J, Weston L, Patel CK. Outpatient Ultra wide-field intravenous fundus fluorescein angiography in infants using the Optos P200MA scanning laser ophthalmoscope. Br J Ophthalmol. 2014;98:302–4.

67. Wu C, Petersen RA, VanderVeen DK. RetCam imaging for retinopathy of prematurity screening. Journal of AAPOS: Off publ Am Assoc Pediatr Ophthalmol Strabismus/Am Assoc Pediatr Ophthalmol Strabismus. 2006;10:107–11.

68. Schwartz SD, Harrison SA, Ferrone PJ, Trese MT. Telemedical evaluation and management of retinopathy of prematurity using a fiberoptic digital fundus camera. Ophthalmology. 2000;107:25–8.

69. Roth DB, Morales D, Feuer WJ, Hess D, Johnson RA, Flynn JT. Screening for retinopathy of prematurity employing the retcam 120: sensitivity and specificity. Arch Ophthalmol. 2001;119:268–72.

70. Ells AL, Holmes JM, Astle WF, et al. Telemedicine approach to screening for severe retinopathy of prematurity: a pilot study. Ophthalmology. 2003;110:2113–7.

71. Chiang MF, Keenan JD, Starren J, et al. Accuracy and reliability of remote retinopathy of prematurity diagnosis. Arch Ophthalmol. 2006;124:322–7.

72. Ng EY, Lanigan B, O'Keefe M. Fundus fluorescein angiography in the screening for and management of retinopathy of prematurity. J Pediatr Ophthalmol Strabismus. 2006;43:85–90.

73. Lepore D, Molle F, Pagliara MM, et al. Atlas of fluorescein angiographic findings in eyes undergoing laser for retinopathy of prematurity. Ophthalmology. 2011;118:168–75.

74. Purcaro V, Baldascino A, Papacci P, et al. Fluorescein angiography and retinal vascular development in premature infants. J Matern-Fetal Neonatal Med: Off J Eur Assoc Perinat Med, Fed Asia Ocean Perinat Soc, Int Soc Perinat Obstet. 2012;25(Suppl 3):53–6.

75. Zepeda-Romero LC, Oregon-Miranda AA, Lizarraga-Barron DS, Gutierrez-Camarena O, Meza-Anguiano A, Gutierrez-Padilla JA. Early retinopathy of prematurity findings identified with fluorescein angiography. Graefe's Arch Clin Exp Ophthalmol = Albrecht von Graefes Archiv fur klinische und experimentelle Ophthalmologie. 2013;251:2093–7.

76. Yokoi T, Hiraoka M, Miyamoto M, Kobayashi Y, Nishina S, Azuma N. Vascular abnormalities in aggressive posterior retinopathy of prematurity detected by fluorescein angiography. Ophthalmology. 2009;116:1377–82.

77. Yokoi T, Kobayashi Y, Hiraoka M, Nishina S, Azuma N. Evaluation of scleral buckling for stage 4A retinopathy of prematurity by fluorescein angiography. Am J Ophthalmol. 2009;148(544–50):e1.

78. Henaine-Berra A, Garcia-Aguirre G, Quiroz-Mercado H, Martinez-Castellanos MA. Retinal fluorescein angiographic changes following intravitreal anti-VEGF therapy. Journal of AAPOS: Off publ Am Assoc Pediatr Ophthalmol Strabismus/Am Assoc Pediatr Ophthalmol Strabismus. 2014;18:120–3.

79. Hoang QV, Kiernan DF, Chau FY, Shapiro MJ, Blair MP. Fluorescein angiography of recurrent retinopathy of prematurity after initial intravitreous bevacizumab treatment. Arch Ophthalmol. 2010;128:1080–1.

80. Hu J, Blair MP, Shapiro MJ, Lichtenstein SJ, Galasso JM, Kapur R. Reactivation of retinopathy of prematurity after bevacizumab injection. Arch Ophthalmol. 2012;130:1000–6.

81. Manivannan A, Plskova J, Farrow A, McKay S, Sharp PF, Forrester JV. Ultra-wide-field fluorescein angiography of the ocular fundus. Am J Ophthalmol. 2005;140:525–7.

82. Fung TH, Muqit MM, Mordant DJ, Smith LM, Patel CK. Noncontact high-resolution ultra-wide-field oral fluorescein angiography in premature infants with retinopathy of prematurity. JAMA Ophthalmol. 2014;132:108–10.

Remote Imaging and Smart Software for ROP Screening

5

Eric Nudleman and Michael T. Trese

Keywords

Retinopathy of prematurity (ROP) · Telemedicine · Screening · Neonatal intensive care unit—NICU · Software

Retinopathy of prematurity (ROP) has been a serious health problem since the 1950s [1, 2]. However, screening has been performed the same way using indirect ophthalmoscopy during the last half of the twentieth century to determine the retinal changes of retinopathy of prematurity [3]. Recently, retinopathy of prematurity has been recognized as a serious health and medical legal issue for the medical community [4–8]. The screening for ROP has become increasingly important as therapies have improved and success rates are now acceptably high with conventional treatment [3, 9, 10].

The screening however remains the key to initiate such treatment in a timely fashion. With the advent of digital imaging and telemedicine, we now are able to perform screening examinations with excellent documentation, medical malpractice protection, and deliver outstanding patient care [11–21]. It is important however that the information be gathered and handled in a fashion that achieves good quality and reduces human error. Currently available, the RetCam 120 is an instrument that can be used to acquire wide-angle digital fundus images [12, 19]. The images are generally gathered by the NICU nurse who is comfortable dealing with the small neonate [22]. The image capturing requires some training, the use of a lid speculum, a lubricating gel, and an understanding of retinal anatomy. Generally, six images are captured: the iris, to show pupil size, which is important in the quality of image that can be gathered due to the ring illumination of the RetCam, the posterior pole—superior, inferior, nasal, and temporal retinal views are captured and sent for reading [18, 23]. (A complete description of this image-capturing technique can be found at the FocusROP.com website.)

The process of ROP is one which generally is complete by 10 weeks after the due date, but the critical treatment parameters are achieved during the first several weeks to months of life. The critical time period for intervention appears to be somewhere between 31 weeks and 50 weeks postmenstrual age [10, 24, 25]. The initial treatment is often instituted during the period of

E. Nudleman (✉)
Department of Ophthalmology, Shiley Eye Institute, University of California, San Diego, 9415 Campus Point Dr. #0946, La Jolla, CA 92093, USA
e-mail: eric.nudleman@gmail.com

M.T. Trese
Eye Research Institute, Oakland University Associated Retinal Consultants, 3535 W. 13 Mile Road, #344, Royal Oak, MI 48073, USA
e-mail: mgjt46@aol.com

© Springer International Publishing AG 2017
Andrés Kychenthal B. and Paola Dorta S. (eds.), *Retinopathy of Prematurity*,
DOI 10.1007/978-3-319-52190-9_5

hospitalization. Following image capturing, the digital image material must be downloaded from the camera at this time using a portable drive. In the future, hopefully this will be improved to a wireless transmission to a computer system that can then upload images to a remote disease management site such as FocusROP.

FocusROP is a HIPAA-compliant remote disease management software program that reduces human error of the reader [26]. The readers themselves, as well as the image-capturing personnel, require training and in many circumstances require examination to certify that they are appropriately knowledgeable in ROP care (OMIC insured ophthalmologists in the USA). Once the images are sent to the website, they can be retrieved anywhere around the world via the Internet. The software contains an algorithm that uses the best care paradigm from clinical research trials for ROP screening and care. The photographic examinations are generally done weekly, although sometimes one-half week examinations are needed. The readers are notified by text messaging that an image set needs reading, which allows rapid interpretation. The children may get one bedside examination prior to being discharged from the hospital depending on demographics and image findings.

Using digital image-handling software, these images can then be compared one against the other by the neonatologist, NICU nurse, the ophthalmologist, and parents to see any intervals changes in the child's retinal vessels. This also allows better coordinated care when expert readers are requested [27]. For the first time, this allows all parties to be dealing with the same data set relative to ROP care. Previously the neonatologist had to take the word of the ophthalmologist for the retinal changes. With this type of documentation, the neonatologist can see for themselves how the eye is advancing and progressing, as can the parents, which can engender a more cooperative spirit relative to the child's follow-up. Many of the problems of retinopathy of prematurity are engendered when the child does not return for proper follow-up care [5, 8]. Having digital imaging allows the patient's

parents to be able to see how the retina is progressing and why the child may need further follow-up and treatment. Another feature of the FocusROP software is that the primary reader can designate an expert to which the image set can be sent and an opinion returned to the primary reader to use in their report to their NICU.

The imaging systems for ROP care today does allow better documentation [16–20]. This documentation however also needs to be archived for 22 years [28], which the FocusROP system can do and many hospitals have the capability of doing this themselves (see Fig. 5.1).

The FocusROP (2.0) software is a smart software image-handling program that attempts to eliminate two areas of human error. The Focus program takes images that are captured by the NICU nurse—a pupil image, a posterior pole image, a temporal nasal image, superior and inferior image. The images are uploaded in a pattern that is familiar to the ophthalmologist and seen in Fig. 5.1. Images are then montaged into a single image that needs to be read or analyzed in addition by the ROP Tool. The algorithm in the FocusROP program determines whether or not a bedside examination is required or if a repeat photographic examination is required.

The errors that are possible are first, the nurse uploading the images into the program to be sent to the FocusROP website. The FocusROP and montaging software is capable of identifying images that were loaded into the wrong location and correcting that to allow proper montaging. The individual images are also available to the reader since the reader wants them in that fashion. The reader can also manipulate the brightness, contrast, and color hue to maximize reading images. The other most common doctor error is that the examination schedule is made too long and the computer program can be set to a time frame that is unable to be changed and is of an appropriate examination schedule given the findings. These systems, coupled with the use of the ROP Tool to give an indication of plus disease [29, 30], allow a very safe examination technique for retinopathy of prematurity screening.

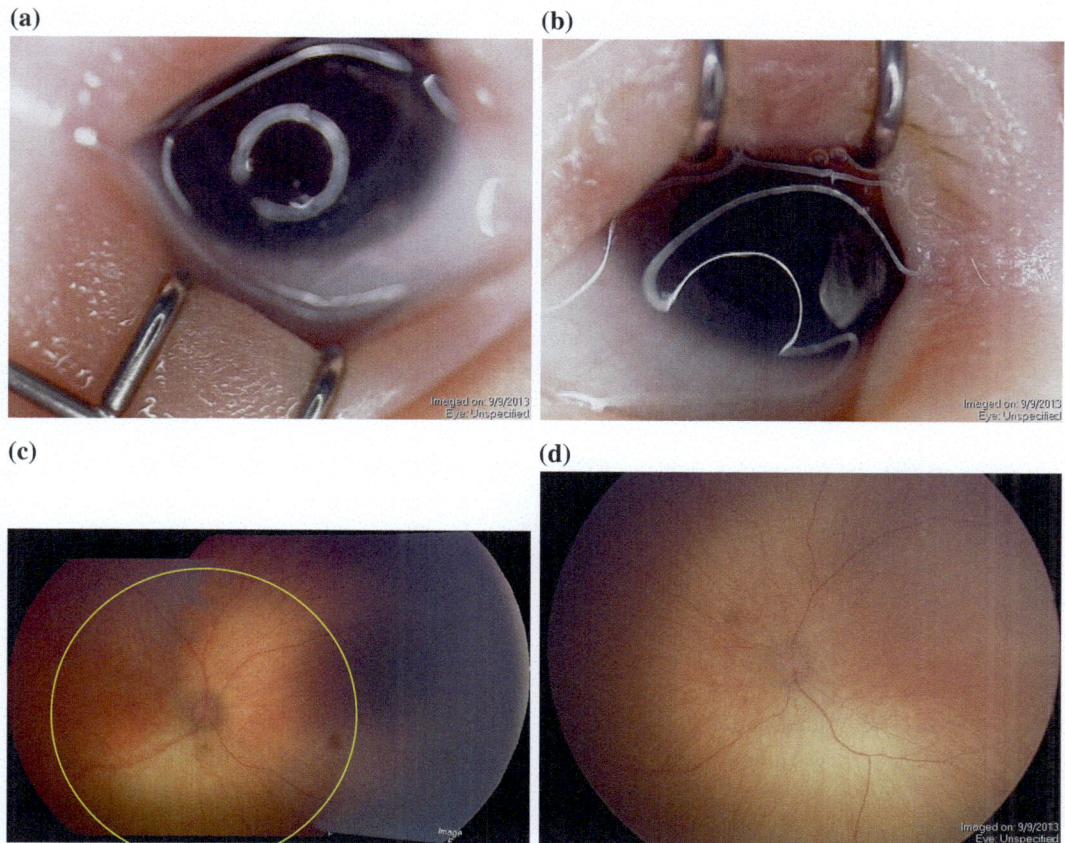

Fig. 5.1 This is a copy of a FocusROP report, which can include images of the retina with Zone 1 drawn or montaged images

It would seem that this type of examination is becoming the standard and the interpretations could be done initially by physicians and non-physician readers, information sent perhaps to the neonatologist who could in fact make the diagnosis based on the information given to them in a safe and reliable fashion, reducing the number of ophthalmology examinations that are needed in the NICU. The role of the non-physician reader has been validated by the EROP Study [31].

Retinopathy of prematurity (ROP) management has changed greatly over the last 20 years and continues to evolve. Currently, with appropriate screening that allows appropriate treatment intervention, the failure rates resulting in blindness for retinopathy of prematurity are reduced to a level of 1–2%, with 90% success of laser [10,

32–35], and 90% success of early lens-sparing vitrectomy [36–40]. The key however to this treatment advantage is appropriate screening. As less than 20% of premature infants with the risk of ROP end up with treatment, it is possible that physicians may be encountering disease at an infrequent rate. Therefore, it may be that the detection of disease is reduced by this infrequent nature of the severe manifestations of retinopathy of prematurity. In many areas of medicine, telemedicine and computer-driven programs are being looked at and used for supplying the physician with information that allows them to make a diagnosis. An example is cardiograms are now often analyzed by computer program giving the physician information that they can use to interpret the patient's cardiogram [41].

It has been known for many years that plus disease is the key change in the fundus which triggers a treatment event [25, 42–44]. A computer program referred to as the "ROP Tool" is a program that gives a number that can be helpful in the determination of plus disease [45]. Plus disease, defined as dilatation and tortuosity in the posterior pole, is something that can be captured, most often quite well, with photographic documentation [29, 46]. The photographs can be analyzed and receive a value based on dilatation and tortuosity. Dilatation is very photographically dependent; whereas, tortuosity can be interpreted by a non-physician reader quite readily [31].

In order to test the hypothesis that the ROP Tool program can match the need for referral-warranted ROP or treatment-warranted ROP, a validation study was designed. Fundus photographs of 335 eyes were read by three experts using the FocusROP software, and then compared to quantitative analysis by the ROP Tool. A scale (0–4) was used by the readers to grade tortuosity. If any photograph was >0, the images were classified as a case. In total, the study included 84 cases and 251 controls. The analysis performed well for identifying tortuosity, but was unable to accurately distinguish dilation in cases from controls. The area under the tortuosity line in a receiver operator curve was 0.918 (95% CI), demonstrating that the ROPtool has a high discriminatory power in differentiating tortuosity between cases and controls (see Fig. 5.1). As a clinical tool, this study demonstrates that the software can provide a sensitive assessment of the need for examination of a child by an ROP expert, potentially reducing cost while delivering quality care.

Virtual Pediatric Retinal Reading Center

The complexity of some forms of pediatric retinal diseases is contributed to by the fact that many of these diseases are rather rare and require a multitude of imaging and diagnostic techniques that are not always easily available to every physician. For that reason, we have established a Pediatric Retinal Reading Center, which can be used to seek advice relative to more complex pediatric retinal issues. These issues include retinopathy of prematurity, pediatric retinal vascular diseases such as familial exudative vitreoretinopathy, persistent fetal vasculature syndrome, Norrie disease, Coats' disease, and other retinal vascular anomalies. Oncology may also be added to this system allowing lesions such as retinoblastoma, retinal hamartomas, and vascular tumors to be evaluated by a group of expert ophthalmologists. This type of electronic consultation is becoming more and more popular and available in a fee-for-service type of package that generates a usable report that can be shared with patients. The access to the Pediatric Reading Center will be available in the first quarter of 2015. The reading center itself may contain some technologies not available in other locations such as use of the ROPtool as has been discussed previously in this chapter. The ability to montage images can allow further analysis of lesion measurements. It also can integrate imaging techniques such as wide-field fluorescein angiography, color fundus photography, optical coherence tomography, and ultrasound. These image sets in the future may also be integrated with genetic findings as more and more genetic information becomes available relative to pediatric retinal diseases. This type of information, since it is available via the Internet, can be delivered to the doctor in a very time efficient fashion after the physician becomes a registered user of the Pediatric Retinal Reading Center service.

The Pediatric Retinal Reading Center can also be used for national and international randomized prospective controlled clinical trials as images can be analyzed and returned to treatment centers in a very rapid fashion globally. A worldwide distribution of information can be gathered that should allow in-depth analysis of what can be very useful information data sets on some diseases that are rare enough that no single physician may be able to accumulate in a meaningful number of patients. The imaging should allow reliable diagnostic information and in some circumstances, the Pediatric Retinal Reading Center may be able to allow entry of vascular active diseases such as retinopathy of prematurity with a description of activity that assures that equally active eyes are being entered into randomized therapeutic selections.

In all, the Pediatric Retinal Reading Center should bring a service to physicians who deal with pediatric retinal diseases and allow them to not function in isolation, but with the support of several other physicians interested in pediatric retinal disease worldwide.

In summary, ROP screening in the twenty-first century involves the team approach of NICU nursing, physician readers, involvement of parents in the long-term care of their child and use of digital imaging and smart software to quantitate the exam. All of these features supply better patient care, mitigates malpractice issues for physicians and hospitals and brings the screening for ROP truly into the twenty-first century using the Internet, which now is so common to manage our banking and social networking, and can also be used to give us ideal patient screening for retinopathy of prematurity. This paradigm results in better medicine, better documentation, and less expense than currently exists for ROP screening.

References

1. Terry TL (1942) Extreme prematurity and fibroblastic overgrowth of persistent vascular sheath behind each crystalline lens. Am J Ophthalmol.
2. King MJ. Retrolental fibroplasia; a clinical study of 238 cases. Arch Ophthalmol. 1950;43:694–711.
3. Fierson WM, American Academy of Pediatrics Section on Ophthalmology, American Academy of Ophthalmology, et al. (2013) Screening examination of premature infants for retinopathy of prematurity. Pediatrics 131:189–195. doi:10.1542/peds.2012-2996.
4. Wang CJ, Little AA, Kamholz K, et al. Improving preterm ophthalmologic care in the era of accountable care organizations. Arch Ophthalmol. 2012;130:1433–40. doi:10.1001/archophthalmol.2012.1890.
5. Demorest BH. Retinopathy of prematurity requires diligent follow-up care. Surv Ophthalmol. 1996;41:175–8.
6. Sims ME. Legal briefs: blindness from retinopathy of prematurity. NeoReviews. 2014;15:e202–5. doi:10.1542/neo.15-5-e202.
7. Simonds M. Management of legal risks associated with the treatment of retinopathy of prematurity. Retinopathy of prematurity. New York, NY: Springer New York; 1992. p. 143–56.
8. Day S, Menke AM, Abbott RL. Retinopathy of prematurity malpractice claims: the ophthalmic mutual insurance company experience. Arch Ophthalmol. 2009;127:794–8. doi:10.1001/archophthalmol.2009.97.
9. Palmer EA, Hardy RJ, Dobson V, et al. 15-year outcomes following threshold retinopathy of prematurity: final results from the multicenter trial of cryotherapy for retinopathy of prematurity. Arch Ophthalmol. 2005;123:311–8. doi:10.1001/archopht.123.3.311.
10. Cooperative FROP (2003) Revised indications for the treatment of retinopathy of prematurity: results of the early treatment for retinopathy of prematurity randomized trial. Archives of ….
11. Schwartz SD, Harrison SA, Ferrone PJ, Trese MT (2000) Telemedical evaluation and management of retinopathy of prematurity using a fiberoptic digital fundus camera. Ophthalmology.
12. Roth DB, Morales D, Feuer WJ, et al. Screening for retinopathy of prematurity employing the retcam 120: sensitivity and specificity. Arch Ophthalmol. 2001;119:268–72.
13. Yen KG, Hess D, Burke B, et al. Telephotoscreening to detect retinopathy of prematurity: preliminary study of the optimum time to employ digital fundus camera imaging to detect ROP. J AAPOS. 2002;6:64–70.
14. Chiang MF, Keenan JD, Du YE, et al. (2005) Assessment of image-based technology: impact of referral cutoff on accuracy and reliability of remote retinopathy of prematurity diagnosis. AMIA Annu Symp Proc 126–130.
15. Lajoie A, Koreen S, Wang L, et al. Retinopathy of prematurity management using single-image vs multiple-image telemedicine examinations. Am J Ophthalmol. 2008;146:298–309. doi:10.1016/j.ajo.2008.04.012.
16. Ells AL, Holmes JM, Astle WF, et al. Telemedicine approach to screening for severe retinopathy of prematurity: a pilot study. Ophthalmology. 2003;110:2113–7. doi:10.1016/S0161-6420(03)00831-5.
17. Lorenz B, Spasovska K, Elflein H, Schneider N. Wide-field digital imaging based telemedicine for screening for acute retinopathy of prematurity (ROP). Six-year results of a multicentre field study. Graefes Arch Clin Exp Ophthalmol. 2009;247:1251–62. doi:10.1007/s00417-009-1077-7.
18. Photographic Screening for Retinopathy of Prematurity (Photo-ROP) Cooperative Group (2008) The photographic screening for retinopathy of prematurity study (photo-ROP). Primary outcomes. Retina (Philadelphia, Pa) 28:S47–54. doi:10.1097/IAE.0b013e31815e987f.
19. Wu C, Petersen RA, Vanderveen DK. RetCam imaging for retinopathy of prematurity screening. J Am Assoc Pediatr Ophthalmol Strabismus. 2006;10:107–11. doi:10.1016/j.jaapos.2005.11.019.

20. Dhaliwal C, Wright E, Graham C, et al. Wide-field digital retinal imaging versus binocular indirect ophthalmoscopy for retinopathy of prematurity screening: a two-observer prospective, randomised comparison. Br J Ophthalmol. 2009;93:355–9. doi:10.1136/bjo.2008.148908.

21. Silva RA, Murakami Y, Lad EM, Moshfeghi DM. Stanford University network for diagnosis of retinopathy of prematurity (SUNDROP): 36-month experience with telemedicine screening. Ophthalmic Surg Lasers Imaging. 2011;42:12–9. doi:10.3928/15428877-20100929-08.

22. Athikarisamy SE, Patole S, Lam GC, et al. Screening for retinopathy of prematurity (ROP) using wide-angle digital retinal photography by non-ophthalmologists: a systematic review. Br J Ophthalmol. 2014;. doi:10.1136/bjophthalmol-2014-304984.

23. Photographic Screening for Retinopathy of Prematurity (Photo-ROP) Cooperative Group, Balasubramanian M, Capone A, et al. (2006) The Photographic screening for retinopathy of prematurity study (Photo-ROP): study design and baseline characteristics of enrolled patients. Retina (Philadelphia, Pa) 26: S4–10. doi:10.1097/01.iae.0000244291.09499.88.

24. Palmer EA, Flynn JT, Hardy RJ, et al. Incidence and early course of retinopathy of prematurity. the cryotherapy for retinopathy of prematurity cooperative group. Ophthalmology. 1991;98:1628–40.

25. Schaffer DB, Palmer EA, Plotsky DF, et al. Prognostic factors in the natural course of retinopathy of prematurity. the cryotherapy for retinopathy of prematurity cooperative group. Ophthalmology. 1993;100:230–7.

26. Faia LJ, Trese MT. Safety net for retinopathy of prematurity management. Expert Review of Ophthalmology. 2010;5:327–31. doi:10.1586/eop.10.9.

27. Chiang MF, Wang L, Busuioc M, et al. Telemedical retinopathy of prematurity diagnosis: accuracy, reliability, and image quality. Arch Ophthalmol. 2007;125:1531–8. doi:10.1001/archopht.125.11.1531.

28. Kraushar MF, Morse PH (2008) Retina and vitreous. In: Springer New York, New York, NY, pp 225–235.

29. Chiang MF, Gelman R, Martinez-Perez ME, et al. Image analysis for retinopathy of prematurity diagnosis. J AAPOS. 2009;13:438–45. doi:10.1016/j.jaapos.2009.08.011.

30. Wittenberg LA, Jonsson NJ, Chan RVP, Chiang MF (2012) Computer-based image analysis for plus disease diagnosis in retinopathy of prematurity. J Pediatr Ophthalmol Strabismus 49:11–9–quiz 10–20. doi:10.3928/01913913-20110222-01.

31. Quinn GE, Ying G-S, Daniel E, et al. Validity of a telemedicine system for the evaluation of acute-phase retinopathy of prematurity. JAMA Ophthalmol. 2014;. doi:10.1001/jamaophthalmol.2014.1604.

32. Iverson DA, Trese MT, Orgel IK, Williams GA. Laser photocoagulation for threshold retinopathy of prematurity. Arch Ophthalmol. 1991;109:1342–3.

33. Laser therapy for retinopathy of prematurity. Laser ROP Study Group. Arch Ophthalmol. 1994;112:154–156.

34. Hunter DG, Repka MX. Diode laser photocoagulation for threshold retinopathy of prematurity. A randomized study. Ophthalmology. 1993;100:238–44.

35. McNamara JA, Tasman W, Brown GC, Federman JL. Laser photocoagulation for stage 3+ retinopathy of prematurity. Ophthalmology. 1991;98:576–80.

36. Capone A, Trese MT. Lens-sparing vitreous surgery for tractional stage 4A retinopathy of prematurity retinal detachments. Ophthalmology. 2001;108:2068–70.

37. Hubbard GB, Cherwick DH, Burian G. Lens-sparing vitrectomy for stage 4 retinopathy of prematurity. Ophthalmology. 2004;111:2274–7. doi:10.1016/j.ophtha.2004.05.030.

38. Moshfeghi AA, Banach MJ, Salam GA, Ferrone PJ. Lens-sparing vitrectomy for progressive tractional retinal detachments associated with stage 4A retinopathy of prematurity. Arch Ophthalmol. 2004;122:1816–8. doi:10.1001/archopht.122.12.1816.

39. Lakhanpal RR, Sun RL, Albini TA, Holz ER. Anatomic success rate after 3-port lens-sparing vitrectomy in stage 4A or 4B retinopathy of prematurity. Ophthalmology. 2005;112:1569–73. doi:10.1016/j.ophtha.2005.03.031.

40. Bhende P, Gopal L, Sharma T, et al. Functional and anatomical outcomes after primary lens-sparing pars plana vitrectomy for Stage 4 retinopathy of prematurity. Indian J Ophthalmol. 2009;57:267–71. doi:10.4103/0301-4738.53050.

41. Willems JL, Abreu-Lima C, Arnaud P (1991) The diagnostic performance of computer programs for the interpretation of electrocardiograms. … England Journal of ….

42. Multicenter trial of cryotherapy for retinopathy of prematurity. Preliminary results. Cryotherapy for Retinopathy of Prematurity Cooperative Group. Arch Ophthalmol. 1988;106:471–479.

43. International Committee for the Classification of Retinopathy of Prematurity (2005) the international classification of retinopathy of prematurity revisited. In: Arch. Ophthalmol. pp 991–999.

44. Davitt BV, Wallace DK (2009) Plus disease. Surv Ophthalmol.

45. Wallace DK, Zhao Z, Freedman SF. A pilot study using "ROPtool" to quantify plus disease in retinopathy of prematurity. J AAPOS. 2007;11:381–7. doi:10.1016/j.jaapos.2007.04.008.

46. Gelman SK, Gelman R, Callahan AB, et al. Plus disease in retinopathy of prematurity: quantitative analysis of standard published photograph. Arch Ophthalmol. 2010;128:1217–20. doi:10.1001/archophthalmol.2010.186.

Aggressive Posterior Retinopathy of Prematurity (APROP)

6

Michael J. Shapiro, Michael P. Blair
and Jose Maria Garcia Gonzalez

Keywords

Retinopathy of prematurity (ROP) · Aggressive posterior retinopathy of prematurity (APROP) · Plus disease · Oxygen-induced retinopathy · Neovascular proliferation · Tunica vasculosa lentis · Bevacizumab · Laser photocoagulation · International classification of retinopathy of prematurity

APROP is an uncommon form of ROP. Untreated, eyes with APROP rapidly progress to retinal detachment and blindness. However, early recognition and prompt treatment often allow for effective management. This chapter updates the category of APROP with a more complete discussion including a detailed description of the features, a range of photographic examples, a discussion of more types of APROP, a treatment of diagnostic challenges, and recognition of earlier APROP in order to increase the opportunities for successful treatment. We also discuss the challenges and the alternatives for its practical treatment in order to improve outcomes.

In 2005 the term APROP was coined and presented as a special form of ROP as part of the revisited International Classification of Retinopathy of Prematurity (R-ICROP) [1]. Before 2005, this severe form of ROP was described rarely and inconsistently, and a variety of terms were used that emphasized particular aspects of the condition: Rush disease [2, 3], zone I ROP [4–7], Fulminate ROP [8, 9], and [Japanese] type 2 ROP [10]. Currently, the descriptive power of the term "APROP" has supplanted all previous terms and remains both the best descriptor and most generally accepted term for this subset of ROP. Therefore, use of the term APROP is most helpful for communication among ROP clinicians and researchers. In this chapter, we join others in the literature and designate as "Classical ROP" (CROP) the more common form of ROP with the typical stages, described in the original ICROP published in 1984 [5, 11–13]. Although described in the original International Classification of Retinopathy of Prematurity (ICROP) [14], we generally rely on the more recent descriptions of CROP in the 2005 R-ICROP because it was better documented using RETCAM imaging.

M.J. Shapiro (✉) · M.P. Blair · J.M.G. Gonzalez
Retina Consultants, LTD, 2454 E. Dempster St.
Suite 400, Des Plaines, IL 60016, USA
e-mail: michaelj.shapiro@gmail.com

M.P. Blair
e-mail: michaelblairmd@gmail.com

J.M.G. Gonzalez
e-mail: jmgarcia451@gmail.com

© Springer International Publishing AG 2017
Andrés Kychenthal B. and Paola Dorta S. (eds.), *Retinopathy of Prematurity*,
DOI 10.1007/978-3-319-52190-9_6

Part 1 Critiques of the R-ICROP Description of APROP

The R-ICROP description of APROP was a landmark. It remains the basic tool for recognition of this very dangerous, yet treatable form of ROP. R-ICROP functioned well to deliver the critical message that APROP was a rapidly progressive and difficult to diagnose condition. Prior to R-ICROP, approximately 25% of the retinal detachments referred to our tertiary ROP practice arose from missed APROP. This declined significantly after the publication and consequently blindness was reduced. Currently, R-ICROP remains the standard description for physicians engaged in the care of acute ROP. However, after 10 years it is time to reevaluate this description.

The major success of the description was its influence on decision-making regarding treatment. After publication of R-ICROP APROP eyes were more effectively treated because the description encouraged the treatment of eyes with "prominence of plus disease" (Fig. 6.1) in the posterior retina without diagnostic equivocation. Once prominent plus was seen, there was no requirement for technical zone 1 location or specific features of stage 2 or 3 in order to diag-

nose APROP. In practice, plus disease became the treatment trigger for treatment. The physician was freed of the burden of documenting stage 3 and could treat eyes with posterior disease that was hard to see or hard to categorize because the term "ill-defined retinopathy" included everything except well-defined CROP. The R-ICROP description caused an attitudinal change that has prevented blindness and is now a fundamental for treatment of APROP. Although later in the chapter we will suggest treatment for additional cases that are destined to become APROP, we strongly support the treatment of all eyes showing prominent plus disease and posterior ROP.

We found two substantive limitations in the R-ICROP description of APROP: First, R-ICROP presents APROP with very heavy emphasis on the severe case, with "prominence of plus disease", which requires immediate treatment. In particular, the statement "can be diagnosed on a single visit and it does not require evaluation over time" essentially applies to the moderately severe and severe disease. In fact, ROP that is destined to become APROP does not arise from CROP. ROP that is destined to reach APROP may often be identified before development of prominent plus disease. The pre-APROP (or early APROP) eye

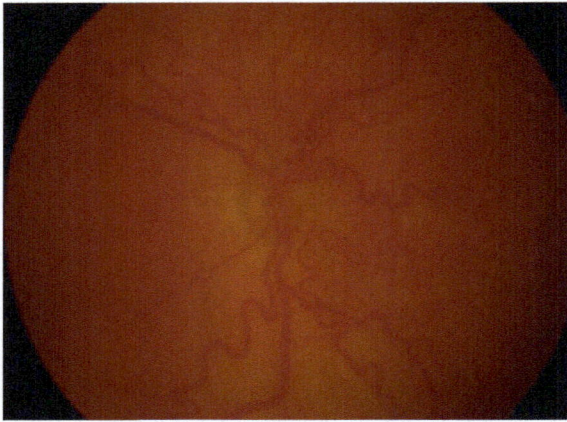

Fig. 6.1 (*Right eye*) Example of prominent plus disease with tortuosity of arteries in four quadrants and venous dilation in four quadrants and venous tortuosity in the nasal quadrant. The nasal quadrants showed more vascular activity with dilation and tortuosity of second- and third-order arterioles and venules than the temporal quadrants. There is no agreed-upon standard for the term prominent plus disease (RETCAM 80 degree lens)

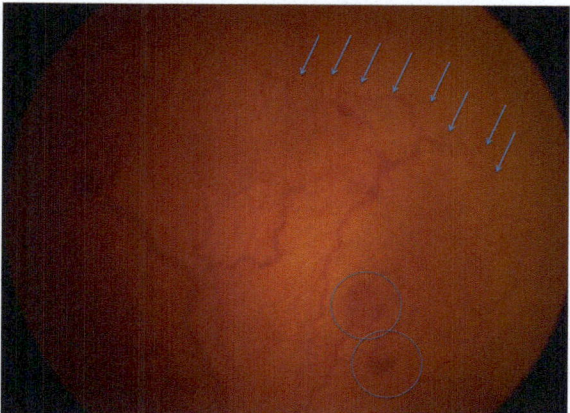

Fig. 6.2 Superior view of *right eye* of the patient seen in Figs. 6.8 and 6.9. A demarcation vessel is seen at arrows. Hemorrhages associated with neovascularization are within circles. Neovascularization appears indistinct as a pink sheet above retinal vessels and obscures details. In this eye, the NV appears slightly posterior to the circumferential vessel

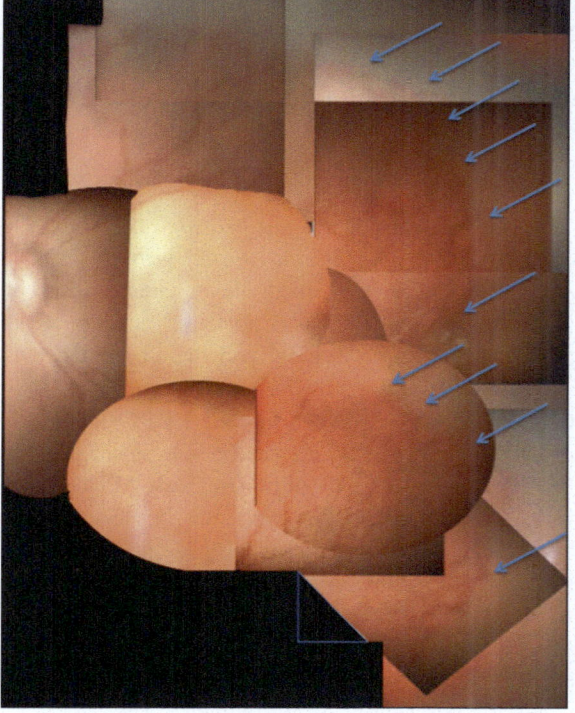

Fig. 6.3 (courtesy of H. Hayashi) Japanese type 2 ROP notes the clear demarcation vessel indicated by a set of long arrows. This is definite APROP despite the absence of posterior plus disease. Evaluated alone, the posterior frame does not show pre-plus

has predictable features that often present with pre-plus and show minimal changes at the vascular–avascular junction or a thin demarcation vessel without distinct neovascularization (Fig. 6.2). Pre-APROP may also present with minimum plus (less than prominent plus) disease and thick demarcation vessels or fine vessel neovascularization (Fig. 6.3). *The lack of recognition in R-ICROP of milder APROP leads to unhelpful delay while waiting for prominent plus disease* [15].

Clinically there is a surprising consequence to this definition. Since the R-ICROP description of APROP required prominent plus disease (Fig. 6.1.), it excluded an APROP equivalent to early treatment of ROP (ETROP) [16] type 1 ROP. For example, there is no equivalent of stage 3 zone I without plus in this definition of APROP. In fact, there is also no true equivalent ETROP type 1 ROP category for APROP stage 2 or 3 with minimum plus, since prominent plus is more than minimal plus and occurs later. Therefore, the ETROP moment for indicated treatment (type 1 or high-risk prethreshold) has no technical APROP equivalent. This diminishes the key contribution of ETROP: that treatment at type 1 ROP had a better response to treatment than the CRYO-ROP threshold ROP. The R-ICROP definition of APROP may result in its being treated later in the disease process closer to CRYO-ROP [17] threshold ROP while CROP is treated at ETROP type 1 ROP. This may contribute to more unfavorable outcomes in eyes with APROP.

Second, *R-ICROP did not provide a distinct category with specific diagnostic criteria of APROP*. ICROP described the characteristic features for APROP as "posterior location, prominence of plus disease, and the ill-defined nature of the retinopathy." However, since posterior location is also seen in zone I CROP and prominence of plus disease can be seen in severe CROP these features do not distinguish APROP from CROP. Moreover, using the description "ill-defined" also did not help identify any specific findings that distinguish the diagnosis of APROP from CROP. Although some examples were provided in the figures, there was no specific criterion to identify retinopathy that meets the description of "ill-defined." This lack has resulted in an APROP literature that is very hard to interpret. It is especially difficult to

interpret articles that lack photographic documentation [18, 19].

Part 2: Practical Diagnosis and Management of APROP

The diagnosis of APROP becomes more helpful when it allows earlier identification and earlier treatment because the response to early treatment improves outcomes as seen in the ETROP study (15). Therefore, the practical objective is to diagnose eyes destined to reach APROP, for example, when plus disease is mild, minimal, or only pre-plus disease is present. For this diagnosis two elements are needed: (1) a reliable positive finding of APROP, when prominent plus disease may not be present; (2) a basis to suspect APROP may be developing.

In our opinion, the most specific positive finding of APROP is neovascularization composed of fine vessels [20] at the border zone between vascular and avascular retina (Figs. 6.2, 6.4, 6.5, 6.6, 6.7, 6.8, 6.9, 6.10, 6.11 and 6.12). Neovascularization is the purely vascular form of fibrovascular proliferation (stage 3). Because of the lack of opaque fibrous elements, the neovascularization may be very low contrast and blend into the background. In the R-ICROP this low contrast neovascularization was referred to as "ill-defined" "deceptive" "featureless" and "modest". This particular language implied that this feature might be easily missed by routine exam. Often, the fine vessels of APROP are not in perfect focus and/or not adequately magnified, therefore, the neovascularization functions as a partially transparent pink overlay that subtly distorts or colors the details of the retina. The transition in color and details may be the key observation. In distinction from the subtlety of APROP, most ROP eyes show high-contrast CROP and the presence of stage 1, 2, or 3 is readily seen with a brief exam. The routine screening exam reflects this reality.

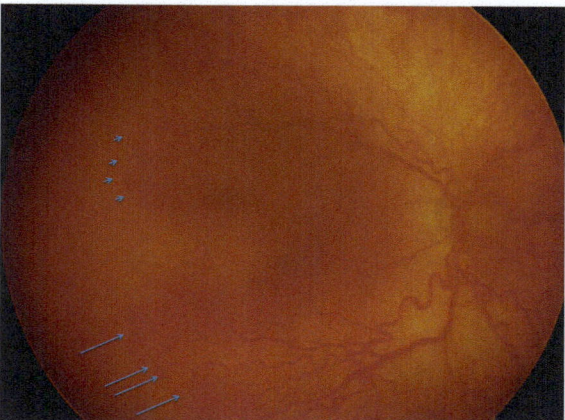

Fig. 6.4 Temporal view of same eye as Fig. 6.1. There is a mild lobular configuration. There is a demarcation vessel (*long arrows*). The fine vessels are not clearly seen temporally but are suspected as the explanation for the increased loss of clear view of blood vessels as one follows the vessels to the periphery indicated by short arrows. Higher magnification and improved focus may be achieved with indirect ophthalmoscope

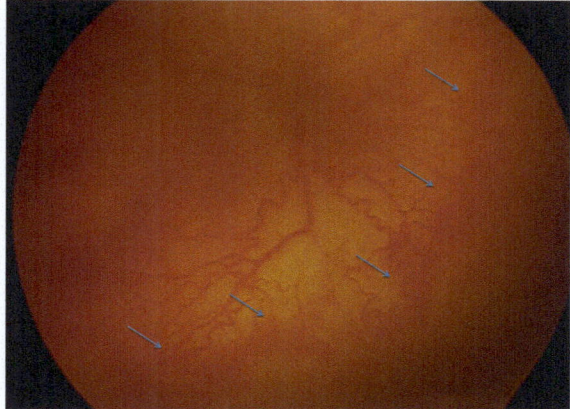

Fig. 6.5 Nasal view of same eye as Fig. 6.1. Prominent plus disease is present. Nasal vessels terminate with a vascular blush that reflects the extensive band of fine neovascularization. *Arrows* denote the posterior border of the neovascular band. Posterior Termination is zone 1. CROP is absent. No foveal reflex is present. A light halo is seen at the posterior edge of avascular retina (Mach Band) without a "definite structure" and is not stage 1 ROP

Unfortunately, this exam routine cannot detect fine vessel neovascularization. In order to detect pre-APROP as a type 1 ROP equivalent, the clinician must take the extra time required to make critical observations. Taking extra time on every exam is burdensome; therefore, identification of APROP suspects is helpful.

We define APROP suspects, as eyes with a mismatch between the clinical picture and the visible ROP stage or with particular red flags described below. Normally young eyes in zone I show attenuated vessels and an involuting hyloidal artery remnant may be detectable. Over time, the vessels dilate to a normal appearance and at that time normal retinal vessel development anteriorly is expected. Eyes with normal caliber and immature vessels in and near zone I must be examined as suspicious, and that suspicion increases if the vessels do not grow anteriorly from week to week. The suspicion is heightened by

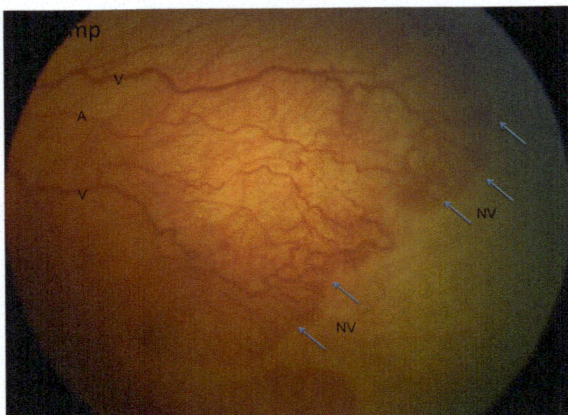

Fig. 6.6 This shows recurrent APROP 11 weeks after injection of bevacizumab. The original diagnosis was APROP and the recurrent neovascularization shows flat brush boarder fronds extending anterior from arteriovenous anastamosis (arrows and NV) without the opaque elements seen in classic stage 1, 2, or 3. (RETCAM 80 degree). The arteriole is marked with a and venule with v. They anastamose behind the fronds

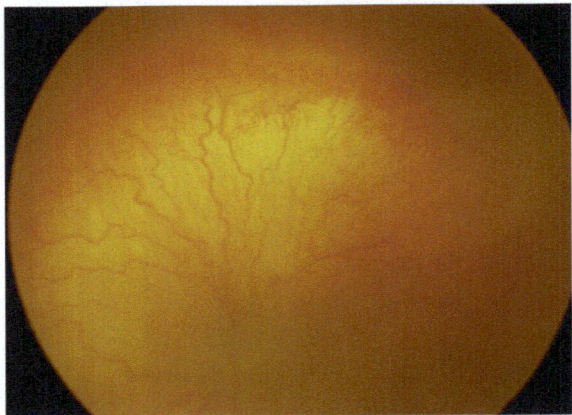

Fig. 6.7 RETCAM 130 image shows a *left eye* with prominent plus disease with arterial and venous tortuosity. Superiorly, an extensive band of neovascular proliferation is seen as a vascular thickening or sheet above the retina that obscures the retinal vessels as they approach the junction of vascular and avascular retina. Again a slight halo, but no definite structure is seen at the edge of the avascular retina (a Mach band). Note dark artifact from small pupil at the *lower right part* of the frame

anterior vascular dilation without CROP stage 1 or stage 2 (Figs. 6.3, 6.4, 6.6, 6.12, 6.13 and 6.14a). Additional, red flags include: (1) annular, c-shaped or arc-shaped hemorrhages that often arise adjacent to neovascularization (Figs. 6.8, 6.9, 6.10, 6.11 and 6.16), (2) retina vessels that lose detail or disappear as they approach the avascular retina (Figs. 6.2, 6.4, 6.5, 6.7, 6.8, 6.9, 6.11 and 6.12), and (3), persistent dilated tunica vasculosa lentis (papillary membrane) (Fig. 6.17).

In most cases, the view of the retina provided by indirect ophthalmoscopy is not ideal for the visualization of fine vessel neovascularization. Detection of similar fine neovascularization in proliferative diabetic retinopathy usually uses higher magnification optical systems than

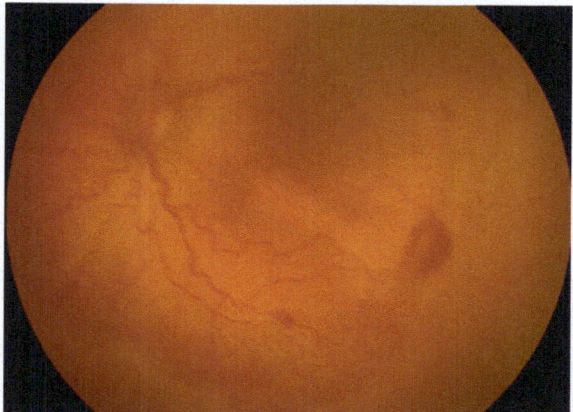

Fig. 6.8 Retcam 130 of *left eye* shows prominent plus disease with tortuosity of arteries and veins. Subtle vascular proliferation is present posterior to the junction. An annular hemorrhage is present. A modest light halo at junction is seen again. Note dark artifact moved to superior temporal area

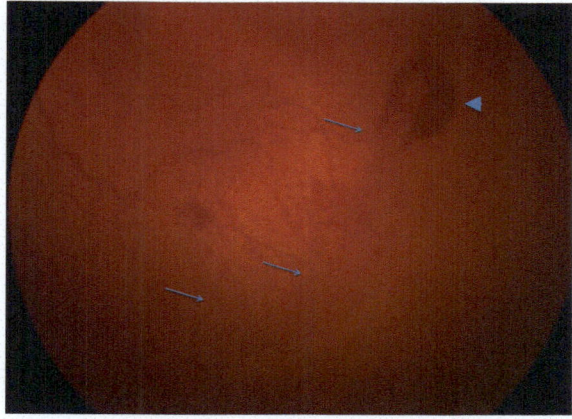

Fig. 6.9 RETCAM 80 degree photograph of the same eye as Fig. 6.8 shows loss of retinal vessel detail approaching the junction since they are obscured by overlying fine vessel neovascularization (especially at *arrows*). Hemorrhage surrounding an area of new vessels (*arrowhead*) is demonstrated. The halo seen in the previous photograph is not a definite retinal structure and may represent a Mach band or a change in the choroid. Note the dark artifact seen in Fig. 6.8 of this same eye is reduced in the 80 degree lens view

provided with standard indirect ophthalmoscopy. Therefore, in order to see these fine vessels with an indirect ophthalmoscope, one must employ strategies to improve resolution. They include adequate pupil dilation, clear media, magnification, improved focus, glare reduction, and control of movement. Dilation may require stronger pharmacologic agents. Magnification will require a 20-diopter lens. Glare reduction may require turning off the nursery's overhead lights or sidelights. Focus may require optimization of the working distance and angles of the condensing lens. The infant may need to be moved out of the bassinette onto a flat surface in order to allow proper working distance. Movement blur may require an assistant to hold the baby's head. Taken together these steps require that the clinician slow down in order to include or exclude the fine neovascularization of APROP. Excluding fine vessel neovascularization of APROP requires an excellent quality of exam and pattern recognition that comes with experience.

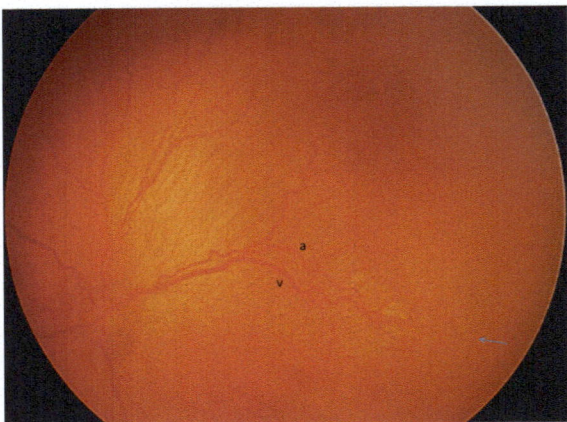

Fig. 6.10 *Left eye* shows a *pink blush* of vascular proliferation posterior at the junction. The vessels posteriorly show pre-plus disease and they remain dilated as they extend to the junction. Following the artery (a) and vein (v) an arterior-venous anastamoses is seen. A frond of vessels grows from anastamosis (*arrow*)

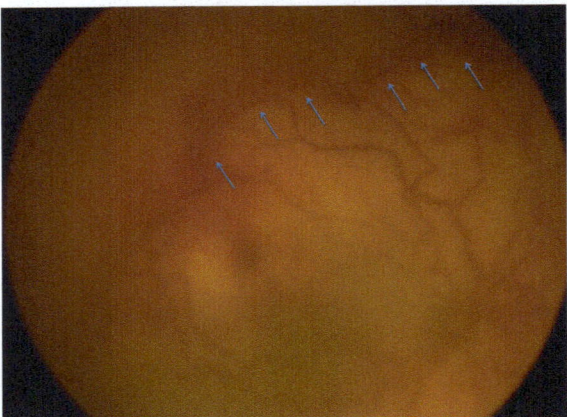

Fig. 6.11 This 80 degree RETCAM image shows prominent plus disease with fine neovascular fronds at the vascular–avascular junction with areas of retina and vitreous hemorrhage. The fronds are elevated into the vitreous (*arrows*). Vitreous hemorrhage contributes to degraded view. Limited depth of field reflect focus above the retina plane

APROP proliferation has a range of appearances and configurations and their recognition can be improved by studying photographs. Many photographs were included with this chapter and more are available at our blog (URL: http://aprophelp.blogspot.com). Studying these photographs may also enhance the examiners pattern recognition of neovascularization and suspicious findings associated with APROP. Review of the text and photos in R-ICROP is also recommended; however, we consider two of the photos in R-ICROP at a later stage of APROP than ideal for a good structural outcome.

Since in APROP, CROP stage 1 and stage 2 are not displayed, APROP may appear to transform from immature to full active APROP. However, APROP is not a transformation but rather a rapid development. The evolution from immature to full form in some cases takes only 2 weeks, which is much faster than CROP. During this developmental interval, examination of posterior vessels will usually show pre-plus disease (Figs. 6.3 and

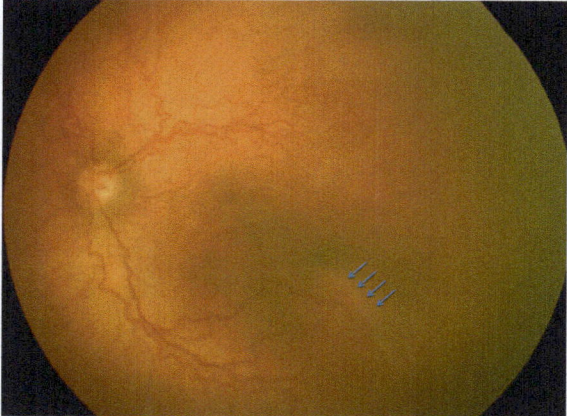

Fig. 6.12 This RETCAM 130 image shows prominent plus disease. The fovea is not vascularized and the vascular retina has a lobular pattern. The flat neovascularization is present and best documented superior temporal but is present around most of the circumference. Inferior temporal there is a white line (*arrows*). This is not CROP stage 1, which is a distinct line in flat retina, but rather fibrous proliferation in an area of vascular contracture causing local retina elevation

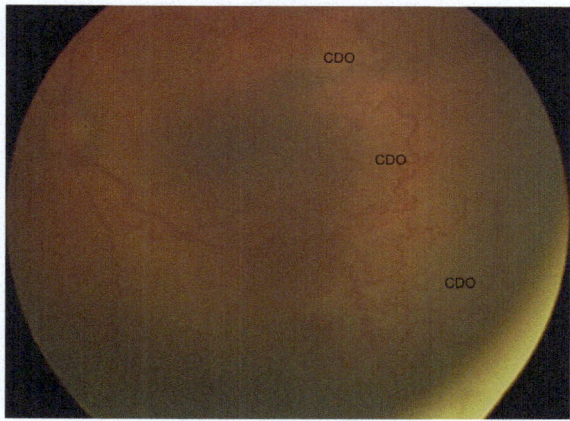

Fig. 6.13 Vascular loops with capillary dropout are a common finding in OIROP found in large babies with uncontrolled oxygen supplementation. This is especially suspicious beyond posterior zone 2. This photo was from a smaller baby but we also suspect an oxygen-induced component when we see this pattern. Liberal oxygen use may occur in infants with concurrent illnesses. CDO labels large areas of capillary dropout surrounded by vascular loops. Prominent dark artifact from small pupil is present using RECAM 130 lens

6.10 and 6.14a). Instead of a line or ridge, the early findings are: (1) vascular dilation posterior to the junction (Figs. 6.10 and 6.14) (this feature may be seen posterior to stage 1 in CROP), (2) posterior intraretinal shunt vessels (Fig. 6.18), (3) limited arteriovenous anastamoses (Figs. 6.6, 6.10 and 6.16) (4) extensive circumferential anastamoses (Figs. 6.4, 6.5 and 6.18), and (5) peripheral shunt vessels (Fig. 6.2 and 6.3). These have also been called demarcation vessels [3]. The retinal vessels may also show general dilation rather than just dilated tips. The circumferential demarcation vessel [21] is a stage 2 equivalent in APROP [3].

In APROP, proliferation starts as a fine frond or network of vessels growing from an anastamosis in the border zone (Figs. 6.3, 6.6, 6.9, 6.10 and 6.11). This neovascularization has been called "flat neovascularization", because it appears flat

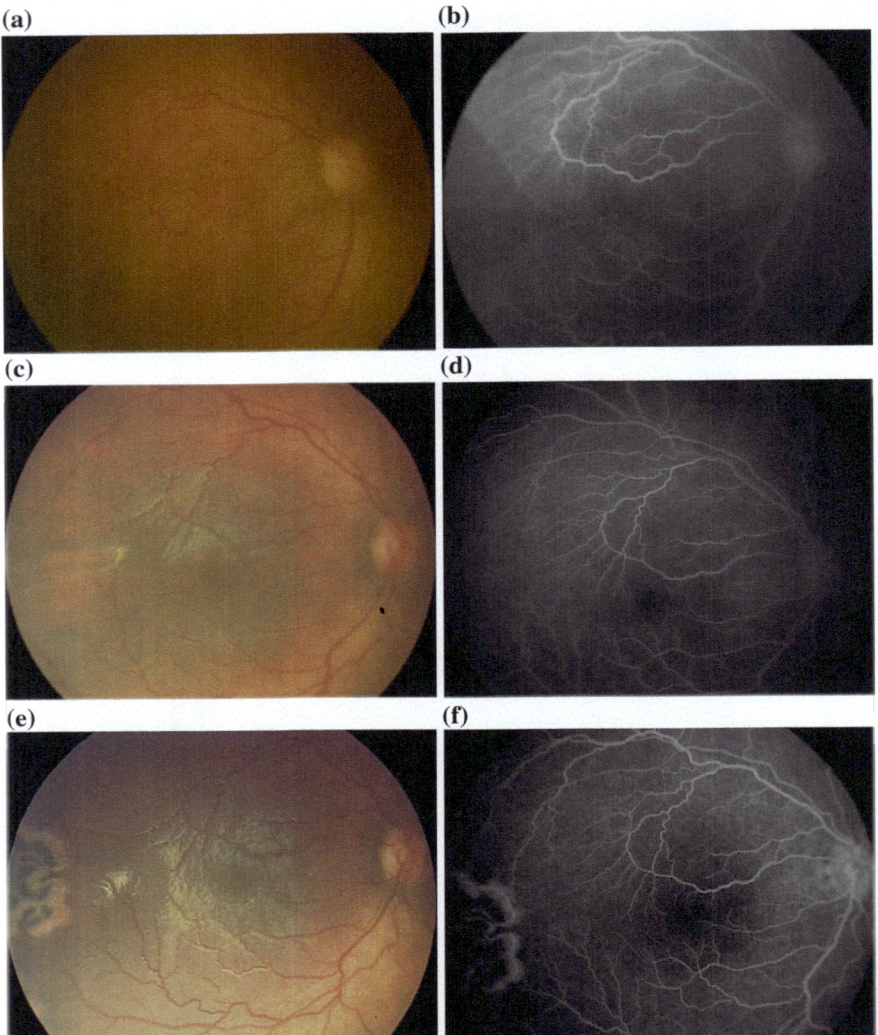

Fig. 6.14 Foveal Vascularization: **a** APROP prior to bevacizumab injection. Note that temporal macula is avascular and foveal vasculature is incomplete. Also note dilated AV shunt superior to fovea. **b** Three weeks and 3 days after bevacizumab injection. Perifoveal vascular ring is nearly complete. **c** Two month and one half months after bevacizumab. Temporal macula is largely vascularized. **d** Fluorescein angiogram shows foveal avascular zone with few microaneurysms. Laser ablation of persistent avascular retina was performed at this visit. **e** Four months after bevacizumab and two months after laser. Foveal depression is seen in center. **f** Fluorescein angiogram shows the perifoveal vascular ring is irregular but clearly present

compared to CROP stage 3. Opaque CROP stage 3 can also give a heightened elevated appearance related to its high contrast. Frequently, APROP proliferation starts as growth along a thin plane above the retina. It also appears especially flat when using the 130-degree RETCAM images. OCT shows it above the retina. In many cases, it will progress by growing anteriorly along the retina and then thicken to become more brush like (Fig. 6.6, 6.10, and also clasic example in blog). The flat pattern is one of the several neovascular configurations. In other eyes the neovascularization grows as a tangle of blood vessels (Fig. 6.2, 6.3, and 6.7). Some photographs show this broad

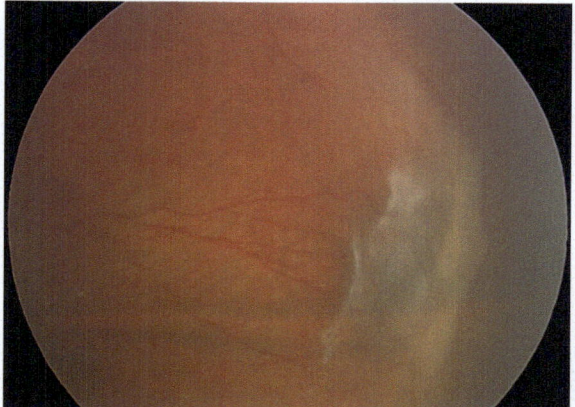

Fig. 6.15 This is cicatricial phase APROP of a flat neovascular network after bevacizumab and subsequent anterior growth of vessels. Untreated APROP will in time gain opaque fibrous elements. This is not CROP stage 2 or three, but rather represents a maturation, opacification, and contraction of the neovascular interstitial tissue and progression toward retinal detachment

Fig. 6.16 Three months after bevacizumab injection posterior recurrence is seen. **a** Shows the color photograph with an anterior ridge areas of round annular and arc-shaped hemorrhages and no plus disease. **b** The angiogram shows the hemorrhages that surround fine vessel neovascularization posterior to a irregularly perfused capillary bed and anterior ridge

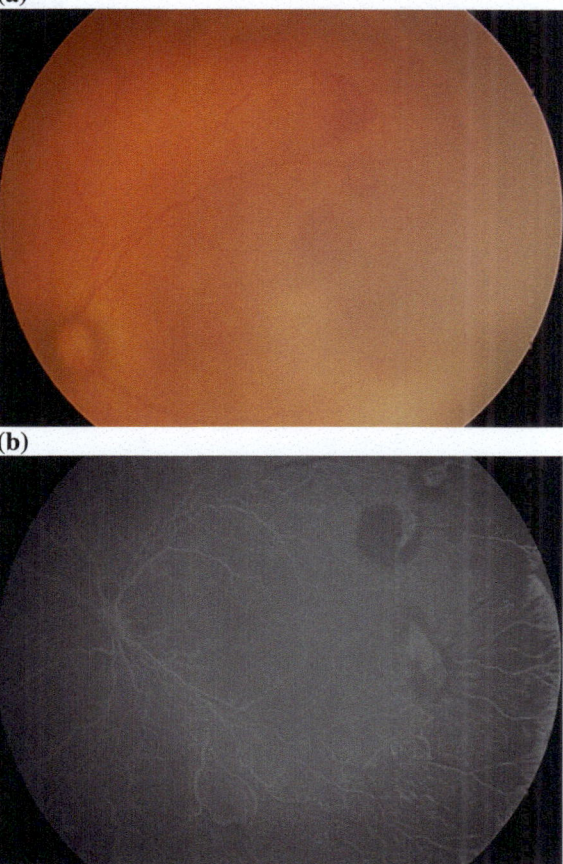

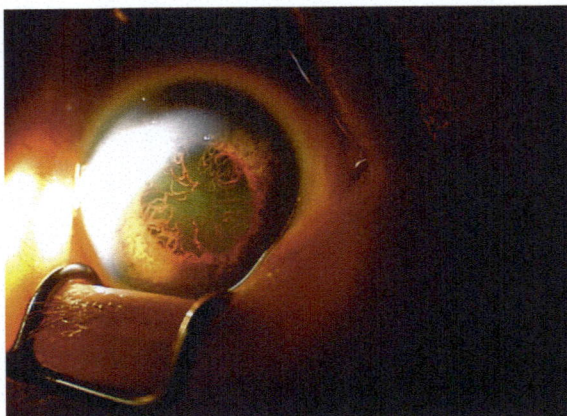

Fig. 6.17 Iris and pupillary membrane vessel engorgement is always accompanied by severe plus disease as defined by the dilation and tortuosity of the retinal vessels. Plus disease with CROP stage 2 or 3 or APROP are indications for treatment. However, this situation reduces the ability to dilate the pupil and to see the details of the retinal pathology. The presence of APROP must be considered regardless of the barriers to examination. Photograph was taken with RETCAM external lens and handheld slit-lamp for illumination

Fig. 6.18 A higher magnification and deeper focus (RETCAM 80) of Fig. 6.5 shows extensive intraretinal shunting posterior to the neovascular band. The *arrow* indicates one example

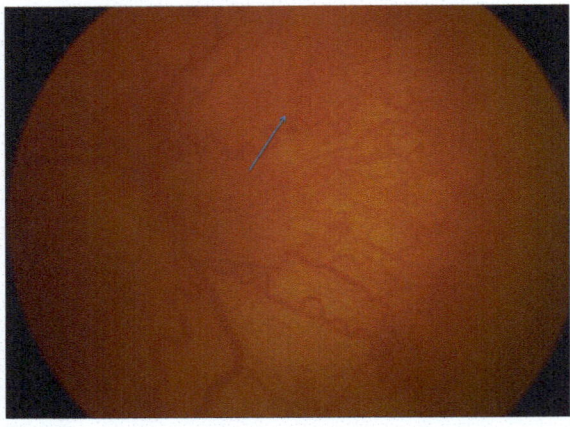

flat growth while others show thickening and extension into vitreous (Figs. 6.7 and 6.11). The fine vessel neovascularization is not required to be flat in order to progress as APROP. As a rule APROP, neovascularization is composed of fine blood vessels and CROP has opaque fibrovascular tissue that ranges from red to light pink. Ultimately both will involute into white fibrous tissue (Figs. 6.12 and 6.15). APROP eyes will progress to involution with a low-contrast, difficult-to-detect neovascular proliferation and detach more quickly. There is a range of neovascularization, and in the R-ICROP description any form of vascular proliferation other than CROP stage 3 (or stage 2 popcorn) is definitive for APROP. However, where R-ICROP requires prominent plus disease, we suggest that feature should not be a prerequisite for all forms of APROP.

After the retina vessels gain moderate plus disease, especially if this is a rapid increase in plus activity, the iris and pupillary vessels may increase in prominence and become reperfused. The hyaloidal arteries may also re-perfuse. Since these vessels may obscure the view of the fundus, the best time to treat is when minimal plus disease appears.

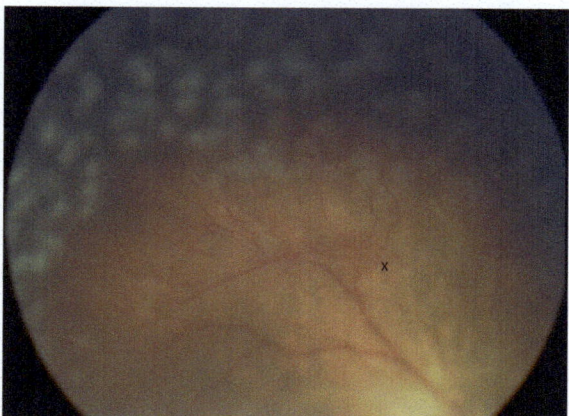

Fig. 6.19 This is a recurrence after injection of bevacizumab. The neovascular proliferation lacks the fibrous
elements and there were no signs of CROP stage 1 or 2 at
the anterior avascular junction. In this case, the
neovascularization is composed of fine vessels that are
low contrast and is seen at the original junction. The
arteriovenous anastomosis is marked with an x and this is
the base of the recurrent neovascularization

Using the RETCAM retinal camera, the
130-degree lens will often not allow high resolution and there is often a prominent central dark
artifact (Figs. 6.8, 6.12, and 6.20). The
130-degree lens best images eyes with blonde
fundus pigmentation. Many of the dramatic
RETCAM advertisements feature blonde fundi.
The 80-degree lens although relatively bulky, is
very helpful in this situation, both for the resolution and for reduction of the central dark artifact. In non-blonde eyes it is essential.
The RETCAM also has little depth of field and
the fine vessels require some fine-tuning in order
to focus the image (Figs. 6.8 and 6.9). The
central dark artifact is plainly present in many
figures included in papers on APROP [13, 17,
22].

Fluorescein angiographic study may also
bridge the gap of low contrast and pupil artifacts
that often lead to poor detail in color RETCAM
photography, and show special features that
when taken with the color photograph are diagnostic. The most important is that fine vessel
neovascularization will be highlighted and show
severe leakage over the course of the angiogram
transit and late phases. The posterior capillary
non-perfusion and abnormalities, and a circumferential vessel may also appear. Eyes with active
pupillary vessels and tunica vasculosa lentis will
leak fluorescein from the anterior segment and
this may degrade the retina vessel study.

Occasionally, vascular loops (Fig. 6.13) are
seen on fluorescein angiography. We interpret
this as loss of capillary perfusion with retention
of larger arterioles and venules. This is different
from a primary defect of angiogenesis and points
to an event of vascular damage such as
oxygen-induced ROP (OIROP). We also expect
some role for the OCT observations on our
understanding of the evolution of APROP and
the effects of treatment. OCT shows neovascular
growth above the retina plane.

In our opinion, APROP fine vessel neovascularization is at least as dangerous as CROP
stage 3 and should be treated using the ETROP
criterion for type 1 ROP and not later. Therefore,
fine vessel neovascularization and minimal plus
disease should be treated with minimum delay in
both zone I and zone II. This is equivalent to
stage 3 with plus and is part of the ETROP
indication for laser treatment. Also, the rare cases
of fine vessel neovascularization without plus
disease in zone I, should be treated as type 1
ETROP. In the ETROP study, eyes showing
stage 2 with plus disease were also treated with
laser. We consider the circumferential demarcation vessel equivalent to stage 2 and when plus
disease is seen with a dilated demarcation vessel,

we think laser treatment should be very strongly considered.

Finally, fine vessel neovascularization and only pre-plus in posterior zone 2 is still a gray situation that we leave to clinical judgment and a case-by-case evaluation. Treatment in cases with definite pre-plus that borders on plus disease may be prudent. However, intensified observation may also be considered in order to catch the moment of mild plus disease. We oppose delay of treatment once plus disease is reached because the risk of blindness far outweighs the ocular risk of treatment in posterior ROP even with mild plus disease. Of course, in this group, which includes seriously unwell infants and requires longer procedures, the systemic risk from stress of the anesthesia and laser treatment requires evaluation by the neonatologist.

We consider these features as additional criteria, because the fine vessels are in fact "ill-defined" "deceptive" "featureless" and "modest", and they are often missed on examinations. Therefore, cases with prominent plus, moderate and severe plus disease, even in the absence of proliferative retinopathy, CROP stage 3 or APROP neovascularization, still require treatment using the plain understanding of the R-ICROP description of APROP. We strongly agree with this established practice and do not demand that the examiner to identify neovascularization before treatment because the most likely reason for not seeing the proliferative retinopathy is a barrier to observation. Severe APROP may be especially difficult to

determine because the anterior segment is often in a high vascular flow state with a dilated persistent vascularized pupillary membrane, tunica vasculosum lentis, or engorged iris vessels (Fig. 6.17). This small pupil is simultaneously a barrier to observation and an important clue for APROP.

In the event that moderate proliferation continues undetected, the next phase in APROP is bleeding from the delicate vessels. Initially, the hemorrhage may appear adjacent or around the neovascularization (Figs. 6.2, 6.8, 6.9 and 6.20) and this is also a strong clue to look for the fine neovascularization. The bleeding is more serious if it extends into the vitreous (Fig. 6.11). Vitreous hemorrhage is a sign of progression toward detachment [23–25]. On the path to retinal detachment, the blood vessels will usually show fibrous tractional elements. These are quite ominous. These cicatricial changes may also be another source of diagnostic confusion. The fibrous tissue may be confused with CROP instead of late APROP (Figs. 6.12 and 6.15)

Part 3: Additional forms of APROP

Oxygen-Induced APROP (Fig. 6.13)

There is a second form of APROP that is critical to recognize. Although it was first beautifully documented in India, it is not limited to India. It has four major distinctions from the first form of APROP [9, 23, 26, 27]. (1) It occurs in situations

Fig. 6.20 A partial c-shaped hemorrhage due to bleeding from the edge of neovascularizarion that was induced after laser, despite a good regression

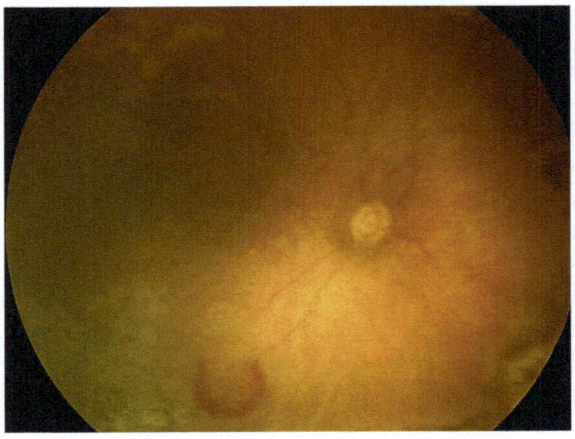

of systemic stress, most commonly the use of unblended, unmonitored, and uncontrolled oxygen supplementation. (2) It occurs among much older infants with gestational age, 28 weeks mean and around 30 weeks median, with birth weights often above 1250 gm. (3) The APROP findings often are not in zone I and may be in mid zone II. (4) The angiogram shows a special pattern of an ablative retinopathy. The ablative pattern shows capillary drop at before loss of larger vessels giving a large vascular looping appearance with dark vascular empty areas in the center. In some more severe cases, the preceding step is also reversed and larger vessels close with hemorrhages of venous stasis and occlusion. This regression of retinal blood vessels increases the extent of non-perfused retina that becomes ischemic. In mild cases, withdrawal of the excessive supplemental oxygen may be helpful or even curative. However, many of these infants will go on to develop proliferation with an APROP fine vascular neovascularization and they need treatment. Another possible difference between OIROP and low gestation APROP is the foveal vasculature, which may develop more normally after OIROP in large older babies since this period of development is farther along when the ROP begins. Finally, as expected, the pattern of vascular retina is not the usual butterfly shape around the nerve. Since capillaries will grow from vascular branches, some notching will occur at the border of the intersecting capillary growth zones.

Oxygen induced retinopathy of prematurity and may occur in developed countries when sick children are treated with high oxygen that induces capillary dropout and vascular involution. This situation was suspected in three cases in South Korea with excellent angiograms [24]. Given that the vascular apical tips are signaled by VEGF and grow forward with capillaries filling in, this peripheral loop pattern probably represents capillary closure rather than selective capillary arrest. The recovery may reflect the persistence of axons that typically lead the vascular development. The pathogenesis of OIROP in human neonates remains uncertain at this time, we hypothesize that this may be the result of

damage from free oxygen radicals and inflammation, and may not be related only to excessive oxygen supplementation alone.

Reactivation   After   Treatment with anti-VEGF (Figs. 6.6, 6.15, 6.19 and 6.16)

We consider it helpful to identify some of the cases of reactivation after prior anti-VEGF treatment as APROP. It shares two major features with APROP. First, fine vessel neovascularization rather than CROP stage 3 has been noted to develop. Second, it is implicated in late unexplained retinal detachments [25]. We remain uncertain if some cases of reactivation with neovascularization might regress with time, but feel that as long as the avascular retina is exposed, systemic stress or another factor may trigger VEGF production and lead to late progression of the retinopathy. As a practical perspective, neovascularization is the prerequisite for retinal detachment and therefore reactivated ROP with neovascularization also poses a risk. When we see fine vessel neovascularization with increasing pre-plus or plus disease, we recommend treatment, either with more anti-VEGF or laser ablation of the avascular zone. Although we lack direct data from a clinical trial, we believe untreated avascular retina is a potential threat. Therefore we treat all significant areas of avascular retina around 55-60 weeks PMA when anesthesia risk is low and long term frequently repeated examination becomes increasingly burdensome.

Mixed ROP
Aside from the early and late cases of APROP, another area of potential confusion arises in eyes with severe plus disease and separate areas of APROP and CROP. For example, some clock hours show brush like neovascularization without any opaque tissue (CROP: stage 1, 2, or 3) while other clock hours show stage 2 ridge structures. Plus disease must be examined by vascular distribution. Each quadrant of plus disease must have a high flow peripheral feature as an explanation for CROP stage 2 or 3 or APROP. The general, the ICROP principle is that

the eye is classified by the most posterior zone and most severe stage. Cases with mixed APROP and CROP, unless there is new data in the future, should be classified into the more severe category, APROP, and treated according to earliest indication.

Unusual Cases

The rare zone II APROP should be examined to detect the end of the retina vasculature as distinct from flat neovascularization. The zone of ROP disease is determined by the end of the retinal vasculature rather than the end of the neovascularization. APROP in zone II should be treated when neovascularization is detected and ablation should include the full avascular zone including the part covered by proliferative retinopathy. Fluorescein angiography may be helpful.

Part 4: Treatment of APROP

APROP is a disease of non-perfusion, ischemia, proliferation, hemorrhage, and traction retinal detachment. The proliferative retinopathy is driven by VEGF. The essence of effective management is the timely reduction of VEGF. Treatment of APROP may be required urgently after the initial exam and efficient diagnosis is essential. Urgent treatment was very dramatically documented in the PHOTO-ROP study in which eyes were treated upon entry [11]. Laser to the complete avascular zone in APROP is markedly less effective than in CROP [13, 21, 28]. Development of retinal detachment in the well-lasered APROP eyes is not infrequent. APROP is also associated with potentially blinding laser complications [29]. In retrospect, APROP-associated treatment failures were a contributor to the poor outcomes of zone I disease in CRYO-ROP. Decades before R-ICROP evidence for the presence of APROP in CRYO-ROP is provided by a photograph in Palmer et.al. Incidence and Early Course of ROP (page 1631) [3] and probably ETROP as well.

The high failure rate after laser treatment for APROP probably reflects both the severity of the disease at diagnosis, and the technical difficulty of complete ablation. The severity of disease may be reduced by recognition of the earlier phase of APROP that are equivalent to type 1 ROP (ETROP study). This earlier treatment time reduces technical challenges. The improvement of the diagnostic exam in order to facilitate detection of earlier phases of APROP was discussed above.

The technical barriers to an excellent laser treatment pattern are: 1. A persistent pupillary membrane (often called a persistent tunica vasculosa lentis) that obscures the retina; 2. Limited field of view from iris rigidity and small pupil from poor dilation and intraoperative constriction; 3. Flat neovascularization may camouflage an underlying area of ischemic retina; 4. Fine neovascularization may be obscured by hazy media; 5. A large area of treatment may increase the risk of laser complication such as inflammation, exudative detachment, ocular ischemia, and cataract; 6. A longer treatment duration and sicker infants may increase the risks of anesthesia. On occasion, these challenges make a complete laser ablation of the avascular retina impossible. Unfortunately, incomplete treatments greatly increase the risk of failure and unfavorable outcome.

In pre-APROP with mild plus disease most of the barriers are mild and laser can be quite effective. Still the laser treatment must include the entire avascular retina including any avascular zones that are under the neovascularization. Since VEGF is largely produce just anterior to the vascularized retina, posterior skip areas have particularly bad outcomes in all cases of ROP especially APROP [11]. When not identified until the disease progresses to include more posterior plus disease, anterior segment vascular engorgement and larger amounts of neovascularization laser become much more challenging and less effective. Moreover, the response to treatment even in cases of perfect and complete laser treatment of the avascular retina may not lead to immediate resolution because of a large reservoir of VEGF in the vitreous. In fact, neovascularization and even detachment may progress despite complete ablation [30]. The plus disease resolution may take 2 or 3 weeks even in cases that are destined to have a good outcome. If one chooses laser, and its implementation is not excellent, one might consider a second session. Azuma describes early vitrectomy in APROP [31]. Practically, we would choose bevacizumab in cases that are "hot" and progressing or not treated to completion especially with posterior skip areas.

In APROP anti-VEGF treatment has a very strong claim for superiority over laser. In the BEAT-ROP study, the only randomized controlled trial of bevacizumab against conventional laser treatment, zone I eyes outcomes were better in the bevacizumab treatment group compared to the laser treatment group [22]. Unfortunately, the BEAT-ROP study did not have a defined group for APROP. Nonetheless it is reasonable to assume that the zone I cases also include APROP cases. Some articles report evidence of effective treatment in APROP as a category; however, they assume a common definition of APROP. We feel the reader cannot assume a specific meaning to this assertion because of the inclusion of ill-defined retinopathy in the R-ICROP definition. The exception is when reports include photographs that allow the reader to confirm the diagnosis directly [32]. In cases with large capillary free zones within the vascularized retina, we believe that OIROP or at least an ablative component must be suspected [33].

The immediate effect of bevacizumab in reversing ROP is quite robust and plainly observed in clinical practice. This qualitative effect has raised important quantitative questions, for example, the optimal dose for the amount of disease (that may treat the estimated VEGF). However, the presence of the effect is noncontroversial. The scientific evidence in favor of the primary treatment with bevacizumab instead of laser is not only the result of a randomized clinical trial (BEAT-ROP), but confirmatory support from a large group of nonrandomized clinical series from around the globe in a variety of populations, all indicating a good reduction in stage 3+ [34]. Although there is little question that the treatment works, a hypothetical concern was raised about potential effects on extraocular tissues during the neonatal and early periods of infant development [35, 36]. This is based on animal models in which complete VEGF blockade is lethal, other animal models with high-dose systemic blockade also describe reduced organ and bone development. In humans and infants, plasma anti-VEGF and prolonged reduction in the systemic VEGF levels were found in the blood after intravitreous injection of bevacizumab [37, 38]. Unfortunately, the clinical relevance is unknown. In the last 8 years, no developmental delays have been linked to the use of intravitreous anti-VEGF. However, recently two papers have claimed to detect neurodevelopmental delays associated with use of intravitreous bevacizumab for ROP in neonates [39, 40]. Neither was randomized and both had presumed bias. The bias arose from selection of more severely affected ROP patients in the bevacizumab group since the severity of ROP is associated with increasing neurodevelopmental risk [41–43].

The biased choice of more severe ROP cases for use of bevacizumab is a widespread effect due to influential opinions promoting special caution in the use of intravitreous bevacizumab. We expect to see increased neurodevelopment deficits in this group with more severe ROP when compared with the unselected patients that received laser. The second major flaw is the use of neurodevelopmental measurements that may not be validated along the full range of visual deficits. Unfortunately, these biases disqualify these papers for use as clinical evidence. At this time without any useful data, it is difficult to assign a weight to the risk and to balance the developmental risk against other risks. Ideally, a long-term and appropriately powered randomized clinical trial would be helpful to allow for scientific evidence. Even an underpowered randomized study may be useful in determining the likelihood of an association, and can later be combined with other studies in future meta-analyses. However, no trial would be adequately powered to completely disprove the hypothesis.

Lack of unequivocal evidence for significant systemic adverse effects requires treating physicians and groups of physicians to make decisions based on clinical judgment. Unfortunately, experience-based clinical judgment is especially subject to decision biases. Among some physicians, the anchoring bias is the serious adverse effects related to other novel ROP treatments. In particular, early reduction of oxygen use for control of ROP has lead to increased mortality [44] and high-dose Vitamin E supplementation increased sepsis [45, 46].

Our perspective recognizes this mixed history of new treatments for ROP and supports effective mechanisms to evaluate the risks. At the conceptual level, the complications from high-dose anti-VEGF given systemically to neonates probably are best approximated by the development of infants with OIROP. In these cases, the oxygen is delivered systemically and is presumed equal in the retina and the rest of the body. The oxygen functions to reduce the VEGF in all tissues. In some of the cases of OIROP, we see dramatic effect on retinal blood vessels. Initially, the capillaries close and then the larger vessels also close. We imagine that such a pattern might occur after an equivalent intravitreous anti-VEGF dosage, but have never seen this vascular closure in patients with our typical dose of 500 micrograms of bevacizumab. Instead, what we have observed after bevacizumab was a regression of neovascularization, a developmental pause, and then a regrowth of fairly normal retinal vasculature. Since the effect in the eye seems qualitatively mild after injection of bevacizumab compared with OIROP, one might assume that the systemic effect from leakage of bevacizumab outside of the eye is also lower after injection of anti-VEGF in the eye compared to systemic oxygen supplementation. Although we suspect that this argument is largely correct, the weakness of this argument is that we do not know how to compare the duration of the two effects and oxygen supplementation probably has a much broader set of direct and indirect target molecules. Also the gestational developmental ages of OIROP and anti-VEGF treatment may be quite different. Finally, in contrast to oxygen that can be dialed up and down, the timeline for biologic activity of the anti-VEGF is probably longer and uncertain.

In situations that have a high risk of blindness with laser treatment, effective bevacizumab treatment is hard to reject without clinical evidence. It seems that only a strong bias can assign greater weight to an unknown, unobserved, uncertain risk over a well-known significant risk. Intravitreous bevacizumab injection has documented risks of infection, cataract, and retinal detachment. In ROP, many centers take efforts to discover complications [47]. The area of uncertainty is the developmental effect. We suspect there may be a relatively small effect that may remain undetectable despite thousands of treatment cases of very prematurely born infants. We expect that cautious and realistic physicians will seriously consider use of bevacizumab in APROP to prevent blindness, not only because of better response of posterior disease to bevacizumab, but also in instances when laser would ablate the fovea (Fig. 6.14). Indeed, bevacizumab as primary treatment in APROP is an increasing trend worldwide because of the higher failure rate of laser in this group [11, 48]. We remain skeptical to both extreme positions: one, that there are no risks to bevacizumab and two, that the risks are common and more severe than blindness.

In our tertiary pediatric practice, the rate of retinal detachment from treatment failure has declined with the use of anti-VEGF either as primary or secondary treatment. The major sources of ROP detachments are now physicians who continue to use laser as primary treatment. We think the rate of failure from laser is still around 10% and most of it was from APROP or high grade CROP. ETROP has eliminated many of the detachments from CROP and anti-VEGF has tremendous potential preventing blindness for much of APROP. Therefore, until there is evidence of substantial counterweighing complications from the treatment, we encourage ROP physicians to use bevacizumab, or other anti-VEGF agents, either as the primary treatment in severe disease and certainly for APROP. It is also reasonable to use the BEAT-ROP criteria for treatment (stage 3+) since they were used in the study population and are structurally more severe than ETROP type 1

ROP, and less severe than CRYO-ROP threshold. If laser is used, we would recommend that pre-APROP that is equivalent to ETROP type 1, be the moment for treatment

We remain vigilant after the use of anti-VEGF because it has a limited blockade effect and a risk of recurrent disease (Figs. 6.6, 6.15, 6.19 and 6.16). These are presumably uncommon and we do not know if they occur in patients with special genetic, inflammatory, or other conditions. Nonetheless, we know some of the patients have late recurrence after anti-VEGF and if untreated this recurrent disease may result in retinal detachment and blindness [25, 48–51]. As a result of these unfavorable outcomes, we are uncomfortable with the prospect of long-term observation of patients showing large residual avascular zones because in most retinal vascular diseases, avascular retina is associated with proliferation, hemorrhage, and retinal detachment. In fact, we suspect based on naturally regressed ROP and FEVR that some recurrences may occur years or even decades later. Therefore, our approach is to treat the acute disease with anti-VEGF and the residual peripheral ischemic retina with laser at a later date.

The retinal detachments after APROP show three patterns. 1. Standard development and location at the border between the vascular and avascular retina. 2. Abnormal location well within the treated avascular zone after apparent regression. 3. Condensed vitreous and fibrous proliferation across the posterior pole with a significant component from anomalous vitreous behavior [38]. APROP may be treated with vitrectomy in early phases to help remove the vitreous reservoir of VEGF. The surgical approach for APROP anomalous vitreous is significantly different from typical retinal detachment after CROP. Likewise detachments limited to the laser treated zone may not be urgent. Vitrectomy after anti-VEGF without peripheral ablation also has other features including an increased risk of dialysis. These topics are beyond the scope of this chapter.

Finally, APROP remains a rare and poorly described form of ROP. We have openly shared our insights and suggested clinical approaches that have evolved from information and experience since the first infant we saw with APROP in 1990 until today. These suggestions remain dynamic and changing and have not been tested by a randomized clinical trial. While we have taken great effort to help the decision-making process for APROP, the suggestions cannot be considered a standard of care.

Appendix: Additional Aspects in the Development of APROP

With detection of early stages of APROP, there are new questions about it natural history. In the era between CRYO-ROP and ETROP, we routinely counted stage 3 clock hours in order to determine presence of threshold ROP. While counting clock hours we also examined eyes at very high risk twice weekly. At that time, the only treatment was laser and eyes without macular development did not undergo subsequent development when it was spared. Initially, we watched a few cases hoping that the fovea would vascularize but it did not. The fastest progression that we observed in APROP neovascular proliferation was about 1 clock hour daily and my sense was that after a 2-week delay APROP was moderate. The neovascularization thickened but remained at the same distance from the optic nerve (Fig. 6.12). Therefore, our opinion based on anecdotal experience with a small number of observed cases, is that there is no ocular advantage in delay of treatment beyond the usual 48 h. We hope for better data in the future. However, we now have a nondestructive alternative to laser treatment. We have seen macular vascularization after treatment with bevacizumab (Fig. 6.14).

Occasionally, there are reports about posterior demarcation lines (stage 1) in APROP [52]. Since we have not seen photographs or an eye with this finding in APROP, it is unclear if this demarcation line is the same or different from the line in ICROP. This finding is not part of R-ICROP as we have understood it. However, in fact if CROP stage 1 is present but stage 2 and 3 do not develop then it meets the R-ICROP "does not progress through the classic stages 1 to 3". This difference points to another area of definitional confusion in APROP, and, therefore, will need to be studied and clarified for the next review of APROP. In any case, the ICROP definition of stage 1 requires more than a halo in order to be called a demarcation line. In ICROP the "line is a thin but definite structure that separates the avascular retina anteriorly from the vascularized retina posteriorly."

Although I have not seen the demarcation line discussed within APROP literature, I assume that my colleagues are reporting a classic stage 1 line. Nonetheless, it is important to be sure this is not a posterior halo, since color contrast is not sufficient to diagnose the presence of a line. Since the perceive color change may reflect a very interesting visual illusion identified by Ernst Mach. This produces an illusion of a line at the border of two shades of gray or color because of the center surround lateral inhibition in the retina. Mach bands are known as a cause for mistaken diagnosis in radiology [53]. This can be true in ROP at the vascular–avascular junction. Many photographs of APROP show a halo at the posterior edge of the avascular retina. Sometimes this changes with reduction of illumination and angle. To add to the confusion of terms in the literature, occasionally the term "demarcation" was used as a noun synonymously for the term "junction" (of the vascularized and avascular retina) [25] (Figs. 6.5, 6.9). Finally, we also wonder if there is yet another halo or demarcation line that may be the result of interstitial fibrous opacification or an edge reflecting marking changes in the choroidal development. Since the posterior retina is very difficult to depress and stereoscopic viewing through small pupil may be limited, the thickness of the stage 1 demarcation line structure cannot always be determined. Finally, we have the impression that the current Japanese ROP literature equates APROP with Japanese type 2 ROP (described and established before R-ICROP) and the two terminologies have evolved in a slightly different manner with communication outcomes that are occasionally at cross purposes (Fig. 6.3).

References

1. International Committee for the Classification of Retinopathy of Prematurity. The international classification of retinopathy of prematurity revisited. Arch Ophthalmol. 2005;123(7):991–9. Review. PubMed PMID: 16009843.
2. Nissenkorn I, Kremer I, Gilad E, Cohen S, Ben-Sira I. 'Rush' type retinopathy of prematurity: report of three cases. Br J Ophthalmol. 1987 Jul;71(7):559–62. PubMed PMID: 3651370; PubMed Central PMCID: PMC1041226.
3. Palmer EA, Flynn JT, Hardy RJ, Phelps DL, Phillips CL, Schaffer DB, Tung B. Incidence and early course of retinopathy prematurity. The cryotherapy for retinopathy of prematurity cooperative group. Ophthalmology. 1991;98(11):1628–40.
4. Katz X, Kychenthal A, Dorta P. Zone I retinopathy of prematurity. J AAPOS. 2000;4(6):373–6.
5. Kychenthal A, Dorta P, Katz X. Zone I retinopathy of prematurity: clinical characteristics and treatment outcomes. Retina. 2006;26(7 Suppl):S11–5.
6. Tasman W. Zone I retinopathy of prematurity. Arch Ophthalmol. 1985;103(11):1693–4. doi:10.1001/archopht.1985.0105011087032.
7. Shapiro MJ, Gieser JP, Warren KA, Resnik KI, Blair NP. Zone I retinopathy of prematurity. In: Shapiro MJ, Biglan AW, Miller M, editors. Retinopathy of prematurity. Proceedings of the international conference on retinopathy of prematurity. Chicago: Kugler Publications, 1993:149–55.
8. Shapiro MJ. Type 2 of Fulminate ROP. In: Kumar H, Shapiro MJ, Azad RV, editors. Apractical approach to retinopathy of prematurity screening and management. New Delhi: Malhotra Enterprises; 2001. p. 23–33.
9. Shah PK, Narendran V, Saravanan VR, Raghuram A, Chattopadhyay A, Kashyap M, Morris RJ, Vijay N, Raghuraman V, Shah V. Fulminate retinopathy of prematurity clinical characteristics and laser outcome. Indian J Ophthalmol. 2005;53(4):261–5. PubMed PMID: 16333175. Shah PK, Narendran V, Saravanan VR, Raghuram A, Chattopadhyay A, Kashyap M, Devraj S. Fulminate type of retinopathy of prematurity. Indian J Ophthalmol. 2004;52(4):319–20. PubMed PMID: 15693324.
10. Uemura Y, Tsukahara I, Nagata M, et al. Diagnostic and therapeutic criteria for retinopathy of prematurity. Committee's Report Appointed by the Japanese Ministry of Health and Welfare. Tokyo, Japan: Japanese Ministry of Health and Welfare; 1974. Japan J. Ophthalmol. 1977;21:366–78.
11. Spandau U, Tomic Z, Ewald U, Larsson E, Akerblom H, Holmström G. Time to consider a new treatment protocol for aggressive posterior retinopathy of prematurity? Acta Ophthalmol. 2013;91(2):170–5. doi:10.1111/j.1755-3768.2011.02351.x Epub 2012 Jan 23.

12. Vinekar A, Trese MT, Capone A Jr. Photographic screening for retinopathy of prematurity (PHOTO-ROP) cooperative group. Evolution of retinal detachment in posterior retinopathy of prematurity: impact on treatment approach. Am J Ophthalmol. 2008;145(3):548–55. doi:10.1016/j.ajo.2007.10.027. Epub 2008 Jan 22. PubMed PMID: 18207120.

13. Shah PK, Narendran V, Saravanan VR, Raghuram A, Chattopadhyay A, Kashyap M, Morris RJ, Vijay N, Raghuraman V, Shah V. Fulminate retinopathy of prematurity—clinical characteristics and laser outcome. Indian J Ophthalmol. 2005;53(4):261–5.

14. The Committee for Classification of Retinopathy of Prematurity. International classification of retinopathy of prematurity. Arch Ophthalmol. 1984;102:1130–4.

15. Woo R, Chan RV, Vinekar A, Chiang MF. Aggressive posterior retinopathy of prematurity: a pilot study of quantitative analysis of vascular features. Graefes Arch Clin Exp Ophthalmol. 2014 Nov 21. [Epub ahead of print] PubMed PMID: 25413261.

16. Early Treatment for Retinopathy of Prematurity Cooperative Group. Revised indications for the treatment of retinopathy of prematurity: results of the early treatment for retinopathy of prematurity randomized trial. Arch Ophthalmol. 2003;121:1684–94.

17. Cryotherapy for Retinopathy of Prematurity Cooperative Group. Multicenter trial of cryotherapy for retinopathy of prematurity. Preliminary results. Arch Ophthalmol. 1988;106:471–9.

18. Gunn DJ, Cartwright DW, Gole GA. Prevalence and outcomes of laser treatment of aggressive posterior retinopathy of prematurity. Clin Experiment Ophthalmol. 2014;42(5):459–65. doi:10.1111/ceo.12280 Epub 2014 Jan 23.

19. Soh Y, Fujino T, Hatsukawa Y. Progression and timing of treatment of zone I retinopathy of prematurity. Am J Ophthalmol. 2008;146(3):369–74. doi:10.1016/j.ajo.2008.05.010 Epub 2008 Jul 7.

20. Schulenburg WE, Tsanaktsidis G. Variations in the morphology of retinopathy of prematurity in extremely low birthweight infants. Br J Ophthalmol. 2004;88(12):1500–3.

21. Drenser KA, Trese MT, Capone A Jr. Aggressive posterior retinopathy of prematurity. Retina. 2010;30 (4 Suppl):S37–40. doi:10.1097/IAE.0b013e3181cb6151.

22. Mintz-Hittner HA, Kennedy KA, Chuang AZ; BEAT-ROP Cooperative Group. Efficacy of intravitreal bevacizumab for stage 3+ retinopathy of prematurity. N Engl J Med. 2011;364(7):603–15. doi:10.1056/NEJMoa1007374. PubMed PMID: 21323540; PubMed Central PMCID: PMC3119530.

23. Shah PK, Narendran V, Kalpana N. Aggressive posterior retinopathy of prematurity in large preterm babies in South India. Arch Dis Child Fetal Neonatal Ed. 2012;97(5):F371–5. doi:10.1136/fetalneonatal-2011-301121 Epub 2012 May 18.

24. Park SW, Jung HH, Heo H. Fluorescein angiography of aggressive posterior retinopathy of prematurity treated with intravitreal anti-VEGF in large preterm babies. Acta Ophthalmol. 2014;92(8):810–3. doi:10.1111/aos.12461 Epub 2014 Jun 9.

25. Hu J, Blair MP, Shapiro MJ, Lichtenstein SJ, Galasso JM, Kapur R. Reactivation of retinopathy of prematurity after bevacizumab injection. Arch Ophthalmol. 2012;130:1000–6.

26. Sanghi G, Dogra MR, Das P, Vinekar A, Gupta A, Dutta S. Aggressive posterior retinopathy of prematurity in Asian Indian babies: spectrum of disease and outcome after laser treatment. Retina. 2009;29 (9):1335–9. doi:10.1097/IAE.0b013e3181a68f3a.

27. Sanghi G, Dogra MR, Katoch D, Gupta A. Aggressive posterior retinopathy of prematurity in infants ≥ 1500 g birth weight. Indian J Ophthalmol. 2014;62(2):254–7. doi:10.4103/0301-4738.128639 PubMed PMID: 24618495.

28. Sanghi Gaurav, Dogra Mangat R, Katoch Deeksha, Gupta Amod. Aggressive posterior retinopathy of prematurity: risk factors for retinal detachment despite confluent laser photocoagulation. Am J Ophthalmol. 2013;155(1):159–64.

29. Gunay M, Sekeroglu MA, Celik G, Gunay BO, Unlu C, Ovali F. Anterior segment ischemia following diode laser photocoagulation for aggressive posterior retinopathy of prematurity. Graefes Arch Clin Exp Ophthalmol. 2014 Aug 9.

30. Suk KK, Berrocal AM, Murray TG, Rich R, Major JC, Hess D, Johnson RA. Retinal detachment despite aggressive management of aggressive posterior retinopathy of prematurity. J Pediatr Ophthalmol Strabismus. 2010;47 Online:e1–4. doi:10.3928/01913913-20101217-06.

31. Nishina S, Yokoi T, Yokoi T, Kobayashi Y, Hiraoka M, Azuma N. Effect of early vitreous surgery for aggressive posterior retinopathy of prematurity detected by fundus fluorescein angiography. Ophthalmology. 2009;116(12):2442–7.

32. Chung EJ, Kim JH, Ahn HS, Koh HJ. Combination of laser photocoagulation and intravitreal bevacizumab (Avastin) for aggressive zone I retinopathy of prematurity. Graefes Arch Clin Exp Ophthalmol. 2007;245(11):1727–30.

33. Ahn SJ, Kim JH, Kim SJ, Yu YS. Capillary-free vascularized retina in patients with aggressive posterior retinopathy of prematurity and late retinal capillary formation. Korean J Ophthalmol. 2013;27(2):109–15.

34. Wu WC, Kuo HK, Yeh PT, Yang CM, Lai CC, Chen SN. An updated study of the use of bevacizumab in the treatment of patients with prethreshold retinopathy of prematurity in taiwan. Am J Ophthalmol. 2013;155(1):150–158.e1. doi:10.1016/j.ajo.2012.06.010. Epub 2012 Sep 8. PubMed PMID: 22967867.

35. Azad R, Dave V, Jalali S. Use of intravitreal anti-VEGF: retinopathy of prematurity surgeons' in Hamlets' dilemma. Ind J Ophthalmol. 2011;59:421–2.

36. Darlow BA, Ells AL, Gilbert CE, Gole GA, Quinn GE. Are we there yet? Bevacizumab therapy for retinopathy of prematurity. Arch Dis Child Fetal Neonatal Ed. 2013;98(2):F170–4. doi:10.1136/

archdischild-2011-301148. Epub 2011 Dec 30. Review. PubMed PMID: 22209748.

37. Sato T, Wada K, Arahori H, Kuno N, Imoto K, Iwahashi-Shima C, Kusaka S. Serum concentrations of bevacizumab (avastin) and vascular endothelial growth factor in infants with retinopathy of prematurity. Am J Ophthalmol. 2012;153(2):327–333.e1. doi:10.1016/j.ajo.2011.07.005. PubMed PMID: 21930258.

38. Wu WC, Shih CP, Lien R, Wang NK, Chen YP, Chao AN, Chen KJ, Chen TL, Hwang YS, Lai CC. Serum vascular endothelial growth factor after bevacizumab or ranibizumab treatment for retinopathy of prematurity. Retina. 2016 Jul 27. [Epub ahead of print] PubMed.

39. Morin J, Luu TM, Superstein R, et al. Neurodevelopmental outcomes following bevacizumab injections for retinopathy of prematurity. Pediatrics. 2016;137(4):e20153218.

40. Lien R, Yu M-H, Hsu K-H, Liao P-J, Chen Y-P, Lai C-C, Wu W-C. Neurodevelopmental outcomes in infants with retinopathy of prematurity and bevacizumab treatment.

41. Msall ME, Phelps DL, DiGaudio KM, Dobson V, Tung B, McClead RE, et al. On behalf of the cryotherapy for retinopathy of prematurity cooperative group. Severity of neonatal retinopathy of prematurity is predictive of neurodevelopmental functional outcome at age 5.5 years. Pediatrics. 2000;106:998e1005.

42. Molloy CS, Anderson PJ, Anderson VA, Doyle LW. The long-term outcome of extremely preterm (<28 weeks' gestational age) infants with and without severe retinopathy of prematurity. J Neuropsychol. 2015 Mar 24. doi:10.1111/jnp.12069. (Epub ahead of print) PubMed PMID: 25809467.

43. Cooke RWI, Hughes LF, Newsham D, Clark D. Ophthalmic impairments at 7 years of age in children born very preterm. Archs Dis Child Fetal Neonatal Ed. 2004;89:F249e53.

44. BOOST II United Kingdom Collaborative Group; BOOST II Australia Collaborative Group; BOOST II New Zealand Collaborative Group, Stenson BJ, Tarnow-Mordi WO, Darlow BA, Simes J, Juszczak E, Askie L, Battin M, Bowler U, Broadbent R, Cairns P, Davis PG, Deshpande S, Donoghoe M, Doyle L, Fleck BW, Ghadge A, Hague W,Halliday HL, Hewson M, King A, Kirby A, Marlow N, Meyer M, Morley C, Simmer K,

Tin W, Wardle SP, Brocklehurst P. Oxygen saturation and outcomes in preterm infants. N Engl J Med. 2013;368(22):2094–104.

45. Phelps DL, Rosenbaum AL, Isenberg SJ, Leake RD, Dorey FJ. Tocopherol efficacy and safety for retinopathy of prematurity: a randomized, controlled, double-masked trial. Pediatrics. 1987;79(4):489–500.

46. Johnson L, Quinn GE, Abbasi S, Otis C, Goldstein D, Sacks L, Porat R, Fong E, Delivoria-Papadopoulos M, Peckham G, et al. Effect of sustained pharmacologic vitamin E levels on incidence and severity of retinopathy of prematurity: a controlled clinical trial. J Pediatr. 1989;114(5):827–38.

47. Jalali S, Balakrishnan D, Zeynalova Z, Padhi TR, Rani PK. Serious adverse events and visual outcomes of rescue therapy using adjunct bevacizumab to laser and surgery for retinopathy of prematurity. The Indian Twin Cities Retinopathy of Prematurity Screening database Report number 5. Arch Dis Child Fetal Neonatal Ed. 2013;98(4):F327–33.

48. Patel RD, Blair MP, Shapiro MJ, Lichtenstein SJ. Significant treatment failure with intravitreous bevacizumab for retinopathy of prematurity. Arch Ophthalmol. 2012;130(6):801–2. doi:10.1001/archophthalmol.2011.1802.

49. Wu W, Yeh P, Chen S, et al. Effects and complications of Bevacizumab use in patients with retinopathy of prematurity. A multicentre study in Taiwan. Ophthalmology. 2011;118:176–83.

50. Moran S, O'Keefe M, Hartnett C, Lanigan B, Murphy J, Donoghue V. Bevacizumab Versus Diode Laser in Stage 3 Posterior Retinopathy of Prematurity. Acta Ophthalmologica. 2014; e406–7. doi:10.1111/aos.12339.

51. Ittiara S, Blair MP, Shapiro MJ, Lichtenstein SJ. Exudative retinopathy and detachment: a late reactivation of retinopathy of prematurity after intravitreal bevacizumab. J AAPOS. 2013;17 (3):323–5. doi:10.1016/j.jaapos.2013.01.004.

52. Yokoi T, Hiraoka M, Miyamoto M, Yokoi T, Kobayashi Y, Nishina S, Azuma N. Vascular abnormalities in aggressive posterior retinopathy of prematurity detected by fluorescein angiography. Ophthalmology. 2009;116(7):1377–82. doi:10.1016.

53. Buckle CE, Udawatta V, Straus CM. Now you see it, now you don't: visual illusions in radiology. Radiographics. 2013;33(7):2087–102. doi:10.1148/rg.337125204. PubMed PMID: 24224600.

Photocoagulation for Retinopathy of Prematurity

Paola Dorta S. and Andrés Kychenthal B.

Abstract

Laser retinal photocoagulation became the main therapeutic option for vision-threatening ROP after it replaced cryotherapy, becoming the standard of care to which all new treatment options should be compared. Although there is a learning curve and it requires appropriate equipment, excellent results can be achieved in the majority of cases with a small proportion of complications.

Keywords

Retinopathy of prematurity (ROP) · Cryo-ROP · Avascular retina · Laser photocoagulation · Early treatment for retinopathy of prematurity (ETROP)

General Considerations

Retinal photocoagulation with a xenon laser was the first technique used for the treatment of active ROP by Nagata in Japan, and it was published in 1968 [1]. Technical difficulties, especially involving the delivery, induced a need to replace therapy by cryo-coagulation [2].

The results of the Cryo-ROP trial in 1988 established that eyes treated with cryotherapy were less likely to become legally blind (44% vs. 62%) and were less likely to have an unfavorable structural outcome. Total retinal detachment still occurred in 22% of treated eyes [3–5].

Despite the initial debates regarding the advantages of laser versus cryotherapy for the treatment of these children, with the advent of more portable laser units, photocoagulation with a laser is currently the treatment of choice. Laser photocoagulation has proven to be even more effective than cryotherapy for threshold disease [6–10]. Local adverse effects can be notorious with cryotherapy in addition to the inferior results obtained with that technique. Today the use of cryo-coagulation can only be considered if there is no possibility of treating with a laser or anti-VEGF drugs depending on the case.

Paola Dorta S. (✉) · Andrés Kychenthal B.
Ophthalmology, KYDOFT Foundation, Av. Luis Pasteur 5280 of 304, Santiago, Chile
e-mail: paoladorta@kydoft.cl

© Springer International Publishing AG 2017
Andrés Kychenthal B. and Paola Dorta S. (eds.), *Retinopathy of Prematurity*,
DOI 10.1007/978-3-319-52190-9_7

It was Landers in 1990 [11] who first described the ablation of the peripheral avascular retina in ROP patients with an argon laser delivered through an indirect ophthalmoscope. Soon after, McNamara [12] showed that laser therapy was as effective as cryotherapy in the treatment of ROP by comparing the efficacy of trans-scleral cryotherapy versus laser photocoagulation delivered by indirect ophthalmoscope in a randomized clinical trial in 22 infants with threshold stage 3+ ROP. Fifteen of 16 eyes randomized to laser therapy and nine of 12 eyes randomized to cryotherapy showed regression.

Additional studies by these and other authors further demonstrated that laser results are comparable to the results of the CRYO-ROP study. Landers [13] treated 15 eyes of nine infants by confluent photocoagulation of the avascular retina using an argon laser via indirect ophthalmoscope. All treated eyes presented at or beyond the threshold of stage 3 retinopathy of prematurity with plus disease. Complete regression was observed in 13 eyes (73%).

In 1992, Fleming [14] and McNamara [15] further reported on the use of a diode laser to treat ROP. Fleming treated nine infants with posterior ROP using the diode laser through an indirect ophthalmoscopic delivery system. Treatment was commenced as soon as plus disease developed. The disease regressed in all eyes. These results were not only positive in terms of ROP treatment, but they also represented early attempts at "pre-threshold" intervention, which later would become the prevailing time for treatment.

McNamara compared trans-scleral cryotherapy with laser photocoagulation in threshold stage ROP in a prospective randomized clinical trial. Twenty-five of 28 eyes of 32 infants treated with diode laser photocoagulation and followed up for at least 3 months underwent regression. Among 24 fellow eyes treated with cryotherapy and followed up for at least 3 months, 20 regressed. A prospective randomized study by Hunter [16] in 1993 performed in 33 eyes that were treated either with diode laser or cryotherapy showed that diode laser peripheral retinal ablation appeared to be as effective as cryotherapy for the treatment of threshold ROP, but it also showed that indirect

diode laser was more convenient: apneic episodes requiring intubation resulted from two cryotherapy sessions but no diode laser sessions; retreatment because of persistent disease was required in cryo-treated eyes only.

In 1993 Preslan [17] reported regression of threshold disease in 16 out 16 eyes in patients treated with an indirect argon laser. Goggin [18] reported on a series of zone II cases using diode lasers obtaining successful outcomes in 81% of 21 eyes. Capone [19] used an indirect diode laser in the treatment of 17 infants (30 eyes) with zone I "threshold" ROP and achieved a favorable outcome in 83.3%.

During the following years these and other publications contributed to a migration from cryo to laser treatment, especially to the use of indirect diode laser systems.

Trans-scleral diode lasers had been successfully used by some authors [20–22], although trans-pupillary retinal photocoagulation with an indirect laser remains the standard of care worldwide. A trans-scleral approach might be used in cases with media opacities [23].

Current Indications for Laser Treatment of ROP

Present indications for peripheral retinal ablation are based on the Early Treatment For Retinopathy Of Prematurity (ETROP) Randomized Trial outcomes. Earlier treatment of eyes with high-risk pre-threshold disease significantly reduced unfavorable visual outcomes from 19.8 to 14.3%, and it decreased unfavorable anatomical outcomes from 15.6 to 9.0%. As a result, earlier treatment is indicated for high-risk pre-threshold disease [24, 25]. Based on the International Classification of ROP (ICROP), an algorithm was developed to identify those infants with high-risk pre-threshold disease who may benefit from earlier treatment, resulting in approximately 8% of screened infants requiring treatment versus 6% by the CRYO-ROP standards.

Type 1 ROP (Zone I any stage with plus, Zone I stage 3 without plus and Zone II stage 2–3

Table 7.1 Current guidelines to treat ROP

Zone I, any stage with plus
Zone I, stage 3 without plus
Zone II, stage 2–3 with plus

with plus) represents those eyes with high-risk disease that would benefit from early treatment, with guidelines stating that treatment should commence within 72 h of diagnosis. Table 7.1 summarizes the recommended early treatment categories.

Type 2 ROP represents those eyes that require close clinical observation for progression but do not require immediate treatment (Zone 1: Stage 1 or 2 without plus disease, Zone 2: Stage 3 without plus disease). These eyes should be considered for treatment only if they progress to type I ROP or threshold.

The final visual acuity results of the ETROP trial showed that at 6 years of age, the early treatment of type 1 eyes resulted in significant improvements in visual acuity, whereas type 2 eyes did not show benefit from early treatment. The application to clinical practice of the above is that Type 1 eyes but not Type 2 eyes should be treated early considering that 52% of Type 2 high-risk pre-threshold eyes would undergo regression of ROP without requiring treatment [26].

Advantages of Laser Versus Cryotherapy

There are several advantages of using lasers instead of cryotherapy to treat ROP. These are summarized in Table 7.2.

McNamara highlighted the advantages of lasers [27] over cryotherapy emphasizing that cryo is stressful on the infant, leaves large scars, and is more difficult for the surgeon to administer. He predicted early that laser therapy was to become the preferred method for treating threshold retinopathy of prematurity because it is easier for the surgeon to administer and is less

traumatic on the infant. Algawi [28] in 1994 was able to demonstrate that eyes with threshold disease treated with diode laser photocoagulation developed significantly less myopia than those treated with cryotherapy. Further studies have also reported that laser photocoagulation provides superior visual acuity and less refractive myopic shift [29–33]. Today, cryotherapy has very limited indications and all efforts should be made to install laser units to treat ROP [33] when peripheral retinal ablation is to be applied.

Tanaka [34] successfully used indirect ophthalmoscope photocoagulation to treat threshold ROP in two premature infants through the transparent wall of an incubator in whom their poor systemic condition would have prevented the use of cryotherapy.

Clearly, laser delivery systems offer advantages over cryotherapy in treating posterior disease. Zone I might be easily reached with a laser but for cryotherapy, conjunctival incisions might be necessary. Nonetheless, it is precisely cases of posterior ROP that remain responsible for the majority of failures of this treatment modality.

A more recent but growing indication is the use of laser photocoagulation of the peripheral retinal in patients who have been treated with anti-VEGF drugs for a posterior disease once the advancing retinal vascularization approaches zone III. This laser application would prevent late recurrences while minimizing the chances of unfavorable results due to loss in the long follow-ups required in these patients. Additionally, this combined treatment modality would still give treated ROP patients the possible benefits of the long-term retinopexy provided by the laser.

Table 7.2 Advantages of laser over cryotheraphy

Less stressful on the infant
Easier to administer
Better structural outcomes
Induces less refractive myopic shift
Provides superior visual acuity

Complications of Laser Treatment for ROP

Both punctate and transient lenticular opacities have been described after indirect retinal photo-coagulation in ROP patients treated with argon [35] and diode lasers [36]. Pogrebniak [37] described a total cataract and Christiansen [38] also described that cataract is a potential vision-threatening complication of argon laser photocoagulation in ROP. Later, in 1998 O´Neil [39] noted that the incidence of cataract formation after argon laser photocoagulation was approximately 1% and may be more likely to occur when persistent hyaloidal vessels are present on the lens.

Other complications included hyphema [40], iris atrophy, hypotony [41], and phthisis [30] most likely secondary to anterior segment ischemia induced by the peripheral ablation with damage to the posterior ciliary arteries [42, 43]. Payse [44] proposed that diode lasers were safer than argon, and they are the recommended type of laser to be used in ROP. To be taken into consideration is that younger postmenstrual age at the time of laser treatment may be related to an increased risk of anterior segment complications [45].

How to Perform Indirect Laser to Treat Type 1 ROP

The treatment can be applied in the neonatal intensive care unit (NICU) or in an operating room, with general anesthesia or with sedation.

The best alternative will depend on many issues regarding the particular setting where the baby is treated. Good communication with the neonatologist and anesthesiologist are essential to choosing the best option for every premature.

An indirect diode laser with a wavelength of 810 nm is the most appropriate. A 28D-condensing lens is suitable although other lenses can be used. Proper sizing of the lid speculum and scleral depressors are also very important.

The baby should be placed in a way that allows the surgeon to clearly view the entire peripheral retina. The surgeon moving along the position of the head of the baby while applying the laser normally helps to attain complete treatment with no skipped areas.

Laser spots should be applied trans-pupillary in a nearly confluent pattern, leaving a space of half to 1 laser spot between adjacent burns over the entire avascular retina (Fig. 7.1). More con-fluent laser treatments would increase the risk of both local and systemic complications. In 2013, Ells [46] proposed additional laser treatment, posterior to the ridge, for eyes with severe stage 3 ROP in zone II (Fig. 7.2). Sixteen out of 18 eyes experienced rapid regression.

Laser burns should produce a dull white lesion. This can be obtained in the majority of cases with a power setting between 150 and 250 mw and a pulse duration of 100 ms. In the areas adjacent to the ridge an increase in the power setting is normally needed. The number of spots can vary greatly between cases, but for a typical zone II case 1000–1500 spots will be needed, whereas for a zone I case the amount of spots can easily increase to over 2000.

Photocoagulation can be performed in repeat mode, but the surgeon must be sure that all spots

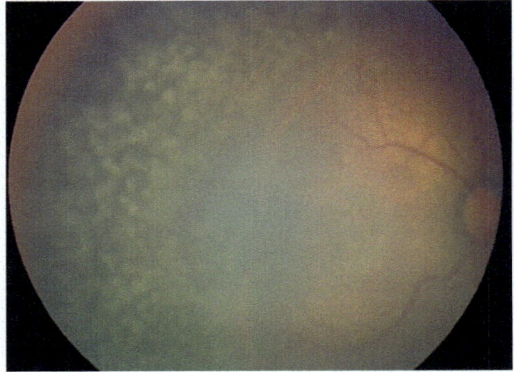

Fig. 7.1 Example of a laser treatment being apply to a type 1 ROP case: laser spots should be applied in a nearly confluent pattern, leaving a space of ½–1 laser spot between adjacent burns over the entire avascular retina

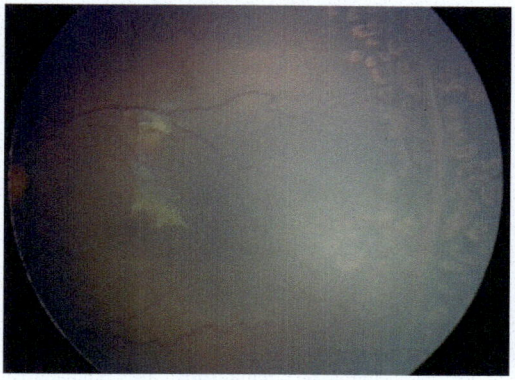

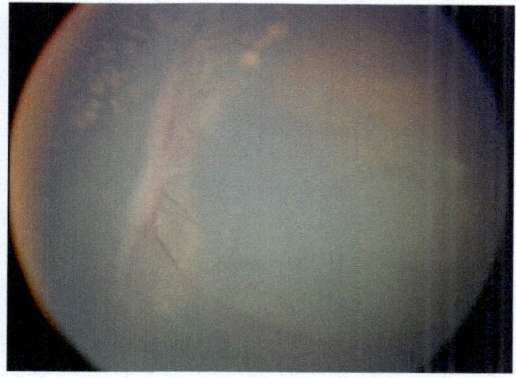

Fig. 7.2 Posterior to the ridge type of laser was applied in this case of severe stage 3 ROP in zone II

Fig. 7.3 Skipped areas can be identified in this case with insufficient laser treatment and progression of the disease

are being applied to the retina. It is advisable to follow an order, starting where the avascular area is greater and then advancing clockwise all around the avascular area until reaching the starting point again. There should be no skipped areas.

Scleral indentation helps to apply the laser in areas closer to the ora serrata. Excessive pressure must be avoided to prevent decompensation of the corneal epithelium and central vein occlusion.

It is important to note that in the first days post-treatment, the disease might continue to progress. Laser photocoagulation acts on the cells that produce VEGF, but it does nothing to the VEGF already present in the eye. Nonetheless signs of regression should be clearly present by 7–10 days after treatment.

Follow-up must be schedule from 48 h post laser treatment in zone I cases to a maximum of 7 days in zone II cases. Patients should then be followed weekly until complete regression. Retreatments are applied in those cases with persistent plus disease or that continue to progress. In this situation, a careful examination should be conducted to find and treat missed or skipped areas (Fig. 7.3).

Laser Photocoagulation in the Anti-VEGF Area

Even with the timing of treatment moved to an earlier stage of the disease by the results of the Early Treatment for Retinopathy of Prematurity (ETROP) study and ablation of the peripheral retina by laser reducing the progression of the disease, patients might still show poor anatomical and visual outcomes after treatment, especially for cases with posterior or zone I disease (Fig. 7.4). Progression to retinal detachment occurred in 12% of eyes in the ETROP study with adequate peripheral ablation.

Vitreal VEGF levels are not reduced by retinal laser photocoagulation and thus might be responsible for the lack of the effectiveness of laser therapy for ROP in some cases. Additionally, laser therapy has some complications including such long-term side effects as a significant decrease in peripheral vision due to ablation of peripheral retina and myopia.

Although there is plenty of evidence to support treating ROP with laser photocoagulation and (depending on the severity) vitreoretinal surgery, there is also an increasing amount of

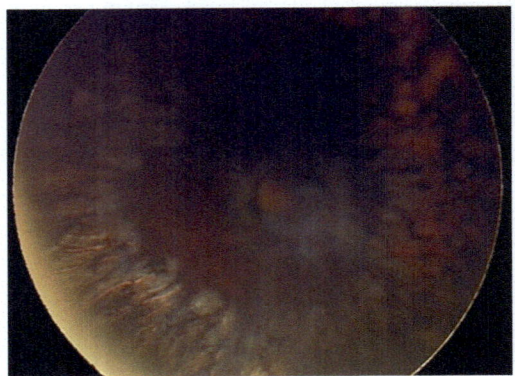

Fig. 7.4 Posterior Zone I case treated with laser. Although effective in avoiding progression to a retinal detachment, limited functional results can be obtained in some of these cases due to the destructive nature of the treatment

clinical work supporting indications for the use of anti-VEGF therapy in some of these patients [47, 48].

Our experience with anti-VEGF drugs in our media supports the use of this treatment as the first-line therapy in cases of zone I ROP. In addition, in posterior Zone I cases without macular development, anti-VEGF can be used shortly after a macula sparing photocoagulation, so as not to risk an unfavorable result due to insufficient laser treatment.

The choice of the treatment modality, either alone or in combination, will depend on many factors in each particular case with the purpose of maximizing the chances of a favorable outcome while minimizing any local or systemic side effects.

References

1. Nagata M, Kobayashi Y, Fukuda H, Suekane K. Photocoagulation for the treatment of retinopathy of prematurity. Jpn J Clin Ophthalmol. 1968;22:419–27.
2. Yamashita Y. Studies on retinopathy of prematurity: III. Cryocautery for retinopathy of prematurity. Jpn J Ophthalmol. 1972;26:385–93.
3. Cryotherapy for Retinopathy of Prematurity Cooperative Group. Multicenter trial of cryotherapy for retinopathy of prematurity. Preliminary results. Arch Ophthalmol. 1988;106:471–9.
4. Cryotherapy for Retinopathy of Prematurity Cooperative Group. Multicenter trial of cryotherapy for retinopathy of prematurity: 3½-year outcome—structure and function. Arch Ophthalmol. 1993;111:339–44.
5. Cryotherapy for Retinopathy of Prematurity Cooperative Group. Multicenter trial of cryotherapy for retinopathy of prematurity: ophthalmological outcomes at 10 years. Arch Ophthalmol. 2001;119:1110–8.
6. Shalev B, Farr A, Repka MX. Randomized comparison of diode laser photocoagulation versus cryotherapy for threshold retinopathy of prematurity: seven-year outcome. Am J Ophthalmol. 2001;132:76–80.
7. Pearce IA, Pennie FC, Gannon LM, et al. Three year visual outcome for treated stage 3 retinopathy of prematurity: cryotherapy versus laser. Br J Ophthalmol. 1998;82:1254–9.
8. O'Keefe M, O'Reilly J, Lanigan B. Longer term visual outcome of eyes with retinopathy treated with cryotherapy or diode laser. Br J Ophthalmol. 1998;82:1246–8.
9. Foroozan R, Connolly BP, Tasman WS. Outcomes after laser therapy for threshold retinopathy of prematurity. Ophthalmology. 2001;108:1644–6.
10. Connolly BP, McNamara JA, Sharma S, et al. A comparison of laser photocoagulation with trans-scleral cryotherapy in the treatment of threshold retinopathy of prematurity. Ophthalmology. 1998;105:1628–31.
11. Landers MB 3rd, Semple HC, Ruben JB, Serdahl C. Argon laser photocoagulation for advanced retinopathy of prematurity. Am J Ophthalmol. 1990;110(4):429–31.
12. McNamara JA, Tasman W, Brown GC, Federman JL. Laser photocoagulation for stage 3+ retinopathy of prematurity. Ophthalmology. 1991;98(5):576–80.
13. Landers MB 3rd, Toth CA, Semple HC, Morse LS. Treatment of retinopathy of prematurity with argon laser photocoagulation. Arch Ophthalmol. 1992;110(1):44–7. Erratum in: Arch Ophthalmol. 1992;110(8):1118.
14. Fleming TN, Runge PE, Charles ST. Diode laser photocoagulation for prethreshold, posterior retinopathy of prematurity. Am J Ophthalmol. 1992;114(5):589–92.
15. McNamara JA, Tasman W, Vander JF, Brown GC. Diode laser photocoagulation for retinopathy of prematurity. Preliminary results. Arch Ophthalmol. 1992;110(12):1714–6.
16. Hunter DG. Repka MX Diode laser photocoagulation for threshold retinopathy of prematurity. A randomized study. Ophthalmology. 1993;100(2):238–44.
17. Preslan MW. Laser therapy for retinopathy of prematurity. J Pediatr Ophthalmol Strabismus. 1993;30(2):80–3.

18. Goggin M, O'Keefe M. Diode laser for retinopathy of prematurity–early outcome. Br J Ophthalmol. 1993;77(9):559–62.

19. Capone A Jr, Diaz-Rohena R, Sternberg P Jr, Mandell B, Lambert HM, Lopez PF. Diode-laser photocoagulation for zone 1 threshold retinopathy of prematurity. Am J Ophthalmol. 1993;116(4):444–50.

20. Seiberth V, Linderkamp O, Vardarli I. Transscleral vs transpupillary diode laser photocoagulation for the treatment of threshold retinopathy of prematurity. Arch Ophthalmol. 1997;115(10):1270–5.

21. Parvaresh MM, Modarres M, Falavarjani KG, Sadeghi K, Hammami P. Transscleral diode laser retinal photocoagulation for the treatment of threshold retinopathy of prematurity. J AAPOS. 2009;13(6):535–8.

22. Parvaresh MM, Falavarjani KG, Modarres M, Nazari H, Saiepour N. Transscleral diode laser photocoagulation for type 1 prethreshold retinopathy of prematurity. J Ophthalmic Vis Res. 2013;8(4):298–302.

23. Trese Michael T. Transscleral photocoagulation to treat ROP in eyes with media opacity. J Ophthalmic Vis Res. 2013;8(4):295.

24. Early Treatment For Retinopathy Of Prematurity Cooperative. Revised indications for the treatment of retinopathy of prematurity: results of the early treatment for retinopathy of prematurity randomized trial. Arch Ophthalmol. 2003;121(12):1684–94.

25. Good WV. Final results of the early treatment for retinopathy of prematurity (ETROP) randomized trial. Trans Am Ophthalmol Soc. 2004;102:233–248, Discussion 248–50.

26. Good WV, et al. Final visual acuity results in the early treatment for retinopathy of prematurity study. Arch Ophthalmol. 2010;128(6):663–71.

27. McNamara JA. Curr Opin Ophthalmol. 1993;4(3):76–80. Laser treatment for retinopathy of prematurity.

28. Algawi K, Goggin M, O'Keefe M. Refractive outcome following diode laser versus cryotherapy for eyes with retinopathy of prematurity. Br J Ophthalmol. 1994;78(8):612–4.

29. Shalev B, Farr AK, Repka MX. Randomized comparison of diode laser photocoagulation versus cryotherapy for threshold retinopathy of prematurity: seven-year outcome. Am J Ophthalmol. 2001;132(1):76–80.

30. Cryotherapy for Retinopathy of Prematurity Cooperative Group. Multicenter trial of cryotherapy for retinopathy of prematurity: natural history ROP: ocular outcome at 5(1/2) years in premature infants with birth weights less than 1251 g. Arch Ophthalmol. 2002;120(5):595–9.

31. Connolly BP, et al. A comparison of laser photocoagulation with cryotherapy for threshold retinopathy of prematurity at 10 years: part 2. Refractive outcome. Ophthalmology. 2002;109(5) 936–41.

32. Ng EY et al. A comparison of laser photocoagulation with cryotherapy for threshold retinopathy of prematurity at 10 years: part 1. Visual function and structural outcome. Ophthalmology 2002;109(5):928–934, discussion 935.

33. Simpson JL, Melia M, Yang MB, Buffenn AN, Chiang MF, Lambert SR. Current role of cryotherapy in retinopathy of prematurity: a report by the American Academy of Ophthalmology. Ophthalmology. 2012;119(4):873–7.

34. Tanaka S. Laser indirect ophthalmoscope photocoagulation in an incubator for the treatment of retinopathy of prematurity. Ophthalmic Surg. 1994;25(1):48–50.

35. Drack AV, Burke JP, Pulido JS, Keech RV. Transient punctate lenticular opacities as a complication of argon laser photoablation in an infant with retinopathy of prematurity. Am J Ophthalmol. 1992;113(5):583–4. Puntual Con argon.

36. Capone A Jr, Drack AV. Transient lens changes after diode laser retinal photoablation for retinopathy of prematurity. Am J Ophthalmol. 1994;118(4):533–5. Puntual Con dido.

37. Pogrebniak AE, Bolling JP, Stewart MW. Argon laser-induced cataract in an infant with retinopathy of prematurity. Am J Ophthalmol. 1994;117(2):261–2.

38. Christiansen SP, Bradford JD. Cataract in infants treated with argon laser photocoagulation for threshold retinopathy of prematurity. Am J Ophthalmol. 1995;119(2):175–80.

39. O'Neil JW, Hutchinson AK, Saunders RA, Wilson ME. Acquired cataracts after argon laser photocoagulation for retinopathy of prematurity. J AAPOS. 1998;2(1):48–51.

40. Simons BD, Wilson MC, Hertle RW, Schaefer DB. Bilateral hyphemas and cataracts after diode laser retinal photoablation for retinopathy of prematurity. J Pediatr Ophthalmol Strabismus. 1998;35(3):185–7.

41. Kaiser RS, Trese MT. Iris atrophy, cataracts, and hypotony following peripheral ablation for threshold retinopathy of prematurity. Arch Ophthalmol. 2001;119:615–7.

42. Lambert SR, Capone A Jr, Cingle KA, et al. Cataract and phthisis bulbi after laser photoablation for threshold retinopathy of prematurity. Am J Ophthalmol. 2000;129:585–91.

43. Ibarra MS, Capone A Jr. Retinopathy of prematurity and anterior segment complications. Ophthalmol Clin North Am. 2004;17(4):577–82.

44. Paysse EA, Miller A, Brady McCreery KM, Coats DK. Acquired cataracts after diode laser photocoagulation for threshold retinopathy of prematurity. Ophthalmology. 2002;109(9):1662–5.

45. Salgado CM, Celik Y, VanderVeen DK. Anterior segment complications after diode laser photocoagulation for prethreshold retinopathy of prematurity. Am J Ophthalmol. 2010;150:6–9.

46. Ells AL, Gole GA, Lloyd Hildebrand P, Ingram A, Wilson CM, Geoff Williams R. Posterior to the ridge laser treatment for severe stage 3 retinopathy of prematurity. Eye (Lond). 2013;27(4):525–30.

47. Dorta P, Kychenthal A. Treatment of type 1 retinopathy of prematurity with intravitreal bevacizumab (Avastin). Retina. 2010;30(Suppl):S24–31.

48. Mintz-Hittner HA, Kennedy KA, Chuang AZ. BEAT-ROP Cooperative Group (2011) Efficacy of intravitreal bevacizumab for stage 3+ retinopathy of prematurity. N Engl J Med. 2011; 364:603–15.

Pharmacomodulation in the Treatment of Retinopathy of Prematurity

8

Khaled Tawansy, Anand Muthiah and Anika Muthiah

Abstract

Type I retinopathy of prematurity is increasing in prevalence proportionate to the advancements of neonatal care and remains the most preventable and potentially devastating neonatal retinal disease worldwide. It is distinguished from standard ROP by its posterior location, aggressive tempo, and high vascular activity/VEGF burden. Current treatment for Type 1 retinopathy of prematurity is guided by landmark multicenter prospective studies (CRYO-ROP, STOP-ROP, ET-ROP, and BEAT-ROP) as well as clinical experience and practical considerations using the available treatment modalities; these include ablation with laser or cryotherapy, intravitreal anti-VEGF agents (Bevacizumab or Ranibizumab) and systemic modulation of hemoglobin and oxygen saturation. Ideal treatment is timed to allow maximum growth of the intrinsic retinal vasculature while preventing fibrovascular contraction or retinal detachment and minimizing complications; these include myopia, visual field constriction, and anterior segment ischemia. With anti-VEGF therapy, recurrences well after the due date and consequent smoldering ROP require vigilant and prolonged outpatient monitoring. Herein, a review of retinal vascular development and the role of VEGF in ROP precedes a discussion of the hallmark studies and a systematic strategy to prevent ROP-associated vision loss while minimizing unnecessary treatments and morbidity to the fragile preemie. We argue that laser is most appropriate for ROP anterior to the equator and smoldering ROP, while intravitreal bevacizumab is more appropriate for posterior disease, especially in highly fragile neonates and situations where follow-up will be reliable.

K. Tawansy (✉)
Children's Retina Institute, 7447 North Figuero
Street, Pasadena, CA 90041, USA
e-mail: ktawansy@gmail.com

A. Muthiah · A. Muthiah
1039 Stony Brook Ct, Claremont, CA 91711, USA
e-mail: mdanand@gmail.com

A. Muthiah
e-mail: anika623@childrensretina.com

© Springer International Publishing AG 2017
Andrés Kychenthal B. and Paola Dorta S. (eds.), *Retinopathy of Prematurity*,
DOI 10.1007/978-3-319-52190-9_8

Keywords
ROP · Techniques · Guidelines · Laser · Anti-VEGF · Dose · Smoldering

Normal Retina and Vasculature

As the most metabolically active tissue in the body, the retina relies on three interrelated circulatory systems; the Hyaloidal Circulation, Choroidal Circulation, and Retinal Circulation. The Hyaloidal vessels emanate from the optic nerve, span the vitreous gel, and surround the crystalline lens and iris (see Figs. 8.1 and 8.2). These vessels perfuse and nourish the entire eye during fetal development, after which they undergo spontaneous apoptosis.

The Choroidal Circulation is a sinusoidal network of blood channels resembling those found in the liver. It bathes the inner sclera, retinal pigment epithelium, and outer retina. Formed by 10 weeks gestation, it is susceptible to compromise by changes in blood pressure and systemic circulation.

The Retinal vessels supply the inner two-thirds of the retina. Growth occurs radially from the optic nerve to the edge of the retina (ora serrata) (see Fig. 8.3), normally arriving at term.

The first phase of normal retinal vascular development occurs from birth to 14 weeks post-conception. This is preprogramed and neural in origin, and is often referred to as the vasculogenesis phase. It is independent of metabolic demands and can be altered by central nervous system disorders. The second phase, angiogenesis, is metabolically driven by a wave of VEGF which leads the path ahead of the

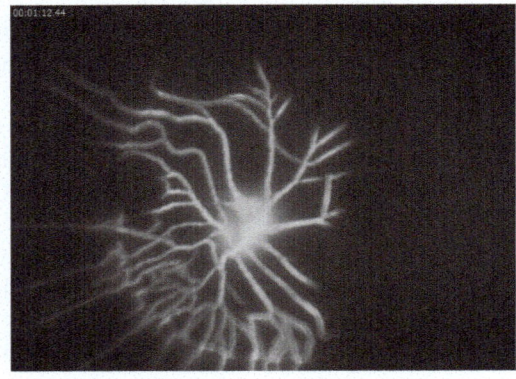

Fig. 8.2 Hyaloidal circulation

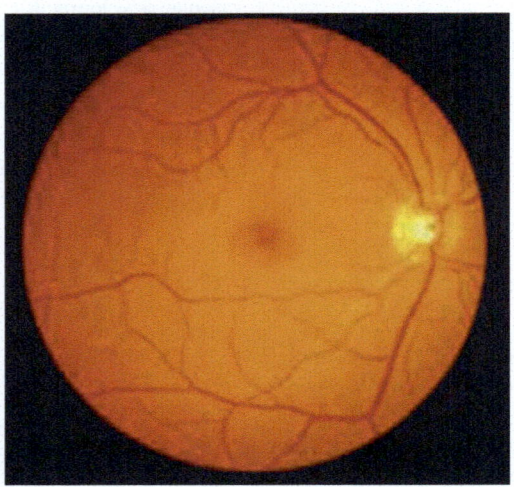

Fig. 8.3 Retinal vessel growth from optic nerve to orra serrata

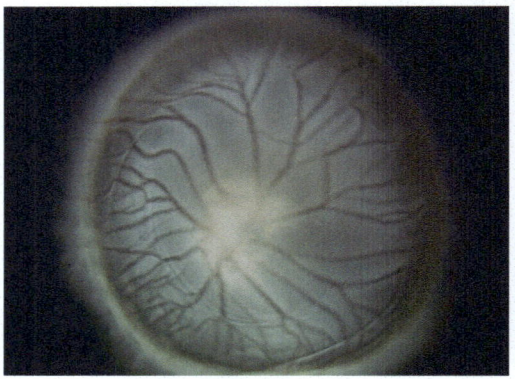

Fig. 8.1 Hyaloidal vessels around the lens

mesenchymal vascular front. Hypoxia is necessary for astrocytes to release this VEGF wave.

Background of ROP

ROP is a bimodal disease that has been linked to excessive oxygen exposure since the early 1950s [1]. An initial phase of vessel loss (vasoobliteration) is followed by a second phase of abnormal new vessel proliferation [2]. Initially discovered as a permeability factor, VEGF was later shown to induce endothelial cell mitosis [3]. VEGF mRNA has been shown to increase with hypoxia and pathologic retinal neovascularization [3–6]. It is now understood that hyperoxia stops normal angiogenesis, leaving an ischemic peripheral retina, which releases supranormal levels of VEGF and IGF-1, the stimuli for extraretinal and sometimes intra-retinal neovascularization [5, 7]. With this overview, the pathophysiology of the two phases of ROP can be understood.

Normal vascularization of the retina begins from the optic disk at 16 weeks gestation and radiates progressively towards the periphery (ora seratta) at 40 weeks post-conception [8]. With premature birth, the normal development of retinal vessels taking place in utero abruptly halts in the setting of relative hyperoxia. The supplemental oxygen given to premature infants leads to a decrease in VEGF levels through a negative feedback loop. The arrest of angiogenesis corresponds to a bump in oxygen saturation from 70% in utero to approximately 99% with respiration of room air. This corresponds to a rise in PaO_2 from 30 mmHg to a range between 60 and 100 mmHg. The primitive vascular bed, in response to the rise in oxygen levels, constricts in an effort to auto-regulate the oxygen. When this constriction persists for four hours or more, it may result in irreversible vasoobliteration.

Phase I ROP takes place from birth to 30 to 32 weeks post conception. As the infant matures, there is an increase in metabolic demands of the retina. High ambient oxygen and consequent vasoobliteration leave the peripheral retina devoid of adequate circulation. This peripheral non-perfused retina becomes hypoxic [2]. With increasing oxygen demand in retinal tissue devoid of circulation, a situation of 'pathologic hypoxia' ensues [1].

Following Phase I vessel loss, pathological neovascularization of the ischemic retina is caused by supranormal quantities of VEGF [1]. Intravitreal injection of anti-VEGF agents has been shown to significantly decrease the neovascular response [9, 10]. Within 24 h of intravitreal injection of 0.625 mg bevacizumab in ROP stage 3 plus, a reliably marked decrease in retinal neovascularization, plus disease, and vessel leakage is demonstrated on fluorescein angiography.

Phase II ROP takes place between 32 and 34 weeks post conception, driven by persistent hypoxia leading to neovascularization. To compensate for ischemia, rapid growth of new vessels occurs at the junction between the vascularized and avascular retina (see Figs. 8.4 and 8.5). Retinal hypoxia is partially compensated by these new vessels, and decreases intrinsic retinal vascular growth through negative feedback [1]. These pathological vessels eventually transform to a fibrovascular cicatrix, which extends from the retina to the vitreous gel and lens. Cicatricial contraction can separate the retina from its pigment epithelium, with ensuing retinal detachment and loss of vision [2].

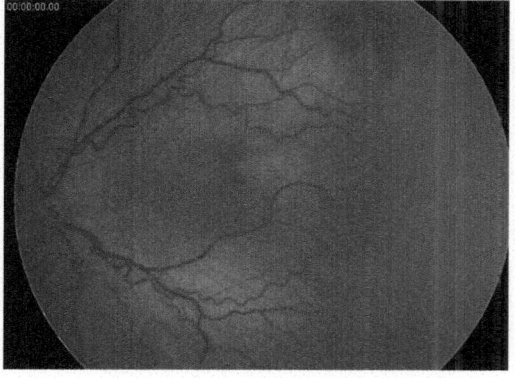

Fig. 8.4 Hypoxia-induced pathologic neovascularization

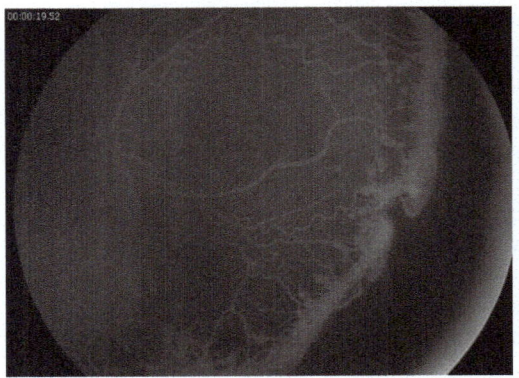

Fig. 8.5 Hypoxia-induced pathologic neovascularization

Standard Versus Aggressive Posterior ROP

Standard or Typical ROP is the most prevalent form of ROP. It typically affects small- to medium-sized preemies under 31 weeks gestation or 1250 g birth weight. Standard ROP follows the typical paradigm of the International Classification of ROP proposed by CRYO-ROP. The timing and progression from stages I to V are predictable, as is the response to ablative treatment.

Type 1 ROP or AP-ROP, is a disease of micro-preemies, who are typically born between 22 and 25 weeks gestation, or very ill older babies. Infants who experience sepsis, acidosis, and unregulated or high fluctuations in O_2 saturations have a greater risk of developing this disease. This is increasing in prevalence as neonatologists with modernized NICUs and O_2 monitoring are sustaining very low birth weight micro-preemies. However, there is also an increase in prevalence in countries that do not have sophisticated NICUs and O_2 monitoring. These populations sustain slightly larger babies that sometimes have unregulated and highly fluctuating O_2 levels that create a form of retinal toxicity. This form of ROP is unfortunately the least understood and is also potentially the most devastating.

AP-ROP is often sinister, moving unpredictably from flat neovascularization to retinal detachment in a matter of days. In the Cryo-ROP study, the majority of retinas with features of AP-ROP progressed to unfavorable structural outcomes, including: retinal detachment, macular folds, and retrolental fibroplasia. The ET-ROP and BEAT-ROP studies were a concerted effort to improve outcomes in cases of AP-ROP [11]. Figure 8.6 is an example of AP-ROP.

Characteristics of AP-ROP include

1. Location in zone 1 and posterior zone 2 as defined by the leading edge of vascular development.
2. Disobeys ICROP classification and can rapidly progress from stage 0 to retinal detachment, within a matter of days or weeks.
3. Very high vascular activity as defined by increased VEGF burden, heavy neovascularization, and prominent tunica vasculosa lentis.
4. A poorly mydriatic stiff iris with neovascularization.
5. Presence of hyphema or vitreous hemorrhage relating to the tendency of the tunica vasculosa lentis and flat or elevated neovascularization to bleed.
6. Aggressive plus disease.

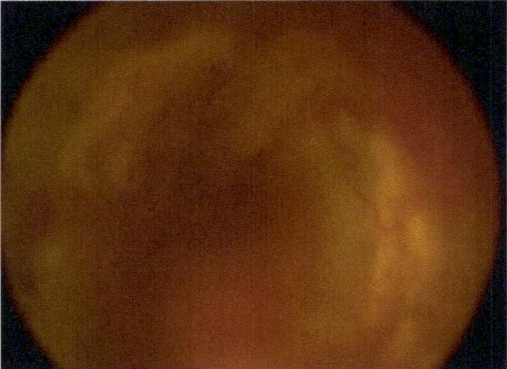

Fig. 8.6 Aggressive posterior ROP

7. Heavy exudates in the vitreous and retina.
8. Massive extraretinal neovascularization.
9. Flat neovascularization.
10. Bizarre patterns of vascular development, sometimes more aggressive nasally than temporally.
11. Requirement for early treatment and multiple treatment sessions to reduce vascular activity.

Smoldering ROP

Typical ROP is a mono-phasic vasculopathy in which threshold for laser ablation occurs in some eyes reliably between 33 and 38 weeks post-conception, and the minority that progress to retinal detachment usually do so within a few weeks after the due date. Traditionally, a child who reaches 45 weeks post-conception without developing pre-threshold features is considered to be at low or no risk for retinopathy of prematurity associated retinal detachment. This concept was first proposed in the Cryo-ROP study.

Cases of ROP progressing to retinal detachment without developing plus disease or pre-threshold characteristics have been observed to occur in the past decade. These eyes have aborted vascular development and are stuck in a state of perpetual non-perfusion and retinal ischemia, otherwise known as Smoldering ROP. Retinal vascular maturation fails to develop, but there is no sufficient VEGF production to create an active shunt and major neovascular proliferation. These eyes are in a non-ending ischemic state and are at risk for developing macular dragging and late retinal detachment, much later than 50 weeks post-conception. In fact, there have been cases of teenagers developing spontaneous tractional detachments after having neonatal ROP that regressed without ablative treatment.

Some of the common characteristics of Smoldering ROP include:

1. A stagnant or fixed leading edge of angiogenesis.
2. Minimal shunt, plus, or neovascularization.
3. Fibrovascular plaque in anterior zone 2 or zone 3.
4. The development of multiple fibrotic concentric ridges, suggesting a stuttering pattern of vascular growth.
5. Circumferential peripheral fibrous traction that can lead to macular dragging, posterior exudation, and a relatively dry retinal detachment.

Prior to the anti-VEGF era this condition was recognized; however its incidence was infrequent. It occurs more often in children with intracranial pathology such as intra-ventricular hemorrhage, microcephaly, periventricular leukomalacia, sepsis, necrotizing enterocolitis, acidosis, high output congenital heart disease, thrombocytopenia, hypoxia, and respiratory distress. Definitive treatment requires semi-confluent ablative laser to the non-perfused zones. This can be guided by fluorescein angiography.

In the anti-VEGF era, Smoldering ROP is being seen with increased frequency in cases that have received anti-VEGF treatment with regression of neovascularization and simultaneous loss of the metabolic drive for vascular development. Cases of late onset retinal detachment after anti-VEGF therapy are largely cases of Smoldering ROP with predominately fibrous proliferation. It is important to recognize this condition and perform ablative treatment when it is clear that intrinsic retinal development has failed. In our practice a "line is drawn in the sand" at the first birthday, which usually corresponds to approximately 75 weeks post-conceptional age. By this time, if the leading edge of vessel development has not reached the ora serrata, in our experience it is unlikely to ever do so. These eyes will remain at risk for fibrous traction/smoldering ROP, potentially for the life of the patient. This risk can be eliminated by semi-confluent laser ablation of the avascular retina, which is best performed using guidance with fluorescein angiography to define zones of non-perfusion.

History of VEGF

In 1948, Michaelson hypothesized that a diffusible angiogenic 'factor X' induced by hypoxia was responsible for iris and retinal neovascularization associated with ischemic retinopathies [12]. This factor was later found to be a glycoprotein vascular permeability factor (VPF) [12]. Independently, in 1989 Leung et al. isolated this same glycoprotein from pituitary follicular cells with characteristics of an endothelial mitogen, labeled vascular endothelial growth factor (VEGF) [12]. Simultaneously, Keck et al. also discovered a tumor-derived factor inducing vascular permeability, and officially named it 'Vascular Permeability Factor' [12]. It was proven subsequently that these factors were in fact all the same 'factor X' originally described by Michaelson [12].

Additional support for the 'factor X' concept comes from studies of primate retinas that developed neovascularization in response to laser photocoagulation [12]. A diffusible VEGF MRNA was implicated as the instigating agent [12]. Furthermore, patients with active pathologic neovascularization consistently have elevated levels of VEGF Mrna comparison to controls [12].

Type 1 ROP—The CRYO-ROP Study

The CRYO-ROP study is still one of the largest ROP studies to have been done, even 30 years later. Although cryotherapy has now been replaced by newer interventions, the landmark study helped establish the framework for ROP treatment strategies and clinical studies employed today. The International Classification Staging System for ROP was used in the CRYO-ROP study as a means to classify the different stages of ROP [13].

In CRYO-ROP, 291 premature infants weighing less than 1251 g with threshold ROP, stage III+ in five contiguous or eight cumulative clock hours, were enrolled. Of these 291 infants, 254 survived [14]. At 15 years of age,

unfavorable ocular structural outcomes defined as posterior retinal folding or worse were judged by study-certified ophthalmologists [14].

The fifteen year outcomes were favorable for typical ROP. In contrast, zone I disease had unfavorable outcomes in approximately 50%. This has led to alternative treatment paradigms as the Multicenter Trial of Cryotherapy of ROP reported statistically significant evidence that ablation of the peripheral nonvascularized retina of premature infants affected with 'threshold' ROP was safe and effective [14]. The question of stability of treatment benefit was answered by the 15-year outcome data of the CRYO-ROP study. Complications of stage III ROP occur decades after treatment, and include: retinal detachment, retinal degeneration, pigment atrophy or migration, cataract, glaucoma, band keratopathy, and hypotony. CRYO-ROP found 30% of treated eyes and 51.9% of control eyes ($p < 0.001$) had unfavorable structural outcomes [14]. Between 10 and 15 years of age, new retinal folds, retinal detachments, or obscuration of the view of the posterior pole occurred in 4.5% of treated and 7.7% of control eyes [14]. Unfavorable visual acuity outcomes were found in 44.7% of treated and 4.3% of control eyes ($P < 0.001$) [14]. CRYO-ROP concluded that near confluent cryo-obliteration may reduce progression of zone 2 threshold ROP to unfavorable structural outcomes. The near confluent treatment may also reduce the need for re-treatment [14].

The ET-ROP Study

ET-ROP explored the possibility of obtaining better structural outcomes by treating high-risk 'pre-threshold' cases of ROP as opposed to waiting until threshold, as done in CRYO-ROP. From the CRYO-ROP experience, the study criteria was developed to identify high-risk cases for early treatment with ablation. High-risk 'pre-threshold' cases were defined as

1. ROP any stage in zone 1.
2. Zone II stage 2 with plus disease.
3. Zone II stage 3 with or without plus disease [11].

Based on patient data from the CRYO-ROP, the ET-ROP study defined high risk as having a $\geq 15\%$ chance of an unfavorable outcome [11]. One eye was kept as a control, it was treated with ablation if threshold was reached.

The 2005 review by the original investigators demonstrated three specific advantages with the early treatment of high-risk pre-threshold ROP cases. The major finding was the reduction in unfavorable visual outcomes occured in the treatment group by 5.5% ($p < 0.005$) [11]. The control eyes of bilateral cases provided additional support as discordant outcomes in two eyes out of 33 infants with bilateral disease; this provided stronger evidence of the beneficial effect of treatment for at high-risk pre-threshold ROP ($P < 0.005$) [11]. Structural outcomes at 9 months provided additional data to support earlier treatment. The treatment group had reduced unfavorable structural outcomes from the 15.6% of conventional treatment group to 9.0%, a 6.6% difference across the groups ($p < 0.001$) [11].

The latest findings published in 2011 showed no statistically significant overall benefit when combining Type I and II cases (18.1 and 22.8% $p = 0.08$) [15]. However, high-risk Type I cases showed a benefit in early treatment compared to control (16.4 vs. 25.2% respectively, $p = 0.004$), and an outcome of 21.3 versus 15.9%, $p = 0.29$ for type II cases [15]. The latest review by the ET-ROP Cooperative Study Group recommends early treatment of Type I eyes, and Type II eyes should be followed closely and without treatment [15].

The pre-threshold types defined by ET-ROP predictably occur between 35 and 37 weeks post-conception. The neovascularization is typically extravascular and responds predictably to standard laser ablation of the avascular retina with a success rate of around 99% when timed appropriately.

The reasoning behind this aggressive stance is that it is difficult to predict which of these cases will have a fulminant course. Although following ET-ROP recommendations may lead to treating significantly more babies than actually necessary, the benefit of reducing unfavorable outcomes requires treating some patients that would have matured well without treatment. ROP is unforgiving in terms of timing, making it difficult to know which cases require treatment. Once ROP accelerates to massive fibrovascular proliferation and cicatricial contraction, the prognosis deteriorates rapidly. ET-ROP advocates 'over treat' some cases in order to prevent any child from losing vision. Systemic complications of early treatment in high-risk pre-threshold cases were greater than conventional including: apnea, bradycardia, and reintubation. One must also consider the ocular implications of treatment and potential secondary effects, which include

1. Constriction of the visual field.
2. High myopia.
3. Inflammatory changes such as synechiae, choroidal effusion, uveitis.
4. Macular pigment alteration.
5. Late onset glaucoma and cataract.
6. Anterior segment ischemia.

Spontaneous Regression Complications

Although ROP is an unforgiving disease, there are instances where regression occurs spontaneously. However, these cases require lifetime follow-up as the following complications may be encountered:

1. Myopia/Anisometropia.
2. Macular dragging.
3. Amblyopia.
4. Cataract.
5. Glaucoma.
6. Late retinal detachment.

The BEAT-ROP Study

BEAT-ROP comparatively studied the outcomes of laser and bevacizumab therapies in 150 infants with bilateral ROP in zone I or posterior Zone II stage 3+ disease [16]. RetCam photography was used to document ROP before randomization; eligibility was established by the treating ophthalmologist and confirmed by a second ophthalmologist on the basis of electronically transmitted RetCam images [16]. One hundred and fifty infants were randomly assigned to two separate groups:

1. Standard confluent laser ablation and fill in for skip areas performed up to 10 days later.
2. Intravitreal injection of Avastin 0.625 mg one dose; a second dose was given for bevacizumab arm recurrences [16].

Cross treatment between groups was not performed as one eye could affect the other. Bevacizumab and VEGF within the circulation and/or substantial inflammation released from laser could confound findings in the other eye and potentially result in irreversible deprivation amblyopia [16].

BEAT-ROP showed an advantage of bevacizumab over ablation in lowering as recurrence 55 weeks. In contrast to CRYO-ROP and ET-ROP, BEAT-ROP looked at recurrence of neovascularization rather than anatomical structure as the primary outcome. (Recurrence of neovascularization in one or both eyes by 54 weeks' postmenstrual age, with ascertainment performed between 50 and 70 weeks) [16].

BEAT-ROP demonstrated the advantage of bevacizumab over laser ablation for Zone I and II as recurrence for the two groups vs 26% (bevacizumab) to 6% (laser) (<0.003) (see Fig. 8.5) [16]. In Zone I alone, the difference was 42 vs 6%. However, the study noted Zone II posterior disease results alone did not differ significantly between both groups [16]. Risk of systemic side effects of bevacizumab could not be determined due to small sample size, so caution is warranted when using this medication in a developing preemie [16].

A review of published literature along with our experiences on this topic failed to disclose a definitive case of systemic toxicity attributable to anti-VEGF therapy in the dose ranges commonly employed. Zone I ablated eyes also reported higher rates of visual field loss, as laser resulted in permanent destruction of vessels and retina while bevacizumab treated eyes demonstrated continued vessel growth into the peripheral retina [16].

Treatment for Typical ROP

First we consider treatment for typical ROP. About two-thirds of cases treated in Southern California have this form of ROP. When the disease is anterior to the equator and the vascular burden is not severe, then it is most reasonable to do semi-confluent laser treatment. One way to lower complications of laser is to treat only anterior to the equator. Because the anterior retina does not serve vision, visual field loss will be minimal. In these cases, we see a very high success rate with minimal complications. As far as timing of treatment, we toe the midline of the CRYOROP and ETROP studies. If there is significant plus disease and a significant burden of stage 2 and 3 disease, then we recommend treatment. Clinical judgement is required to recognize these findings, and this comes with experience. We do not recommend treatment at the first sight of stage 2 plus or 3 plus disease; we reserve treatment until there is a significant degree of vascular activity and ROP burden. Unlike the situation during ET-ROP, we now have the option of anti-VEGF therapy for cases that get too aggressive while under close observation. Because many of these cases will resolve spontaneously, this approach allows us to avoid unnecessary treatment in a significant number of neonates.

Pharmacomodulation Versus Laser

Certain techniques with laser can minimize adverse changes by titrating down the laser energy, doing non-confluent or semi-confluent treatment, or selective/focal laser treatment.

Although ablation is the gold standard and most proven therapy, we are now able to augment this treatment with pharmacomodulation of the eye's biochemistry. The potential advantages with pharmacomodulation of retinovascular development are as follows:

1. It is nondestructive.
2. It changes the aggressive tempo of the disease and takes the pressure off of the treatment timeline.
3. It gives an opportunity for the intrinsic retinal vasculature to develop over time.
4. It can serve as a bridge to take the child from pre-due date to post-due date, which is associated with a change in the biochemistry intrinsically such that VEGF levels go down and TGF-β (antagonistic to VEGF) levels go up.
5. It immediately arrests VEGF activity so that the rapid progression of fibrovascular proliferation to retinal detachment can be aborted more effectively.
6. The results are more rapid than with laser treatment because it immediately soaks up the VEGF in the retina and vitreous cavity.
7. In a critically ill newborn preemie, it is much less stressful to the child to have an injection than having a laser procedure.

Although promising, anti-VEGF therapy has its own constellation of potential problems

a. Possibility of creating infectious endopthalmitis.
b. Traumatizing the lens creating a cataract.
c. Perforating the retina creating a tear or rhegmatogenous detachment.
d. Potential systemic effects on organogenesis at a time when the neonate is very much still developing.
e. Potential optic nerve infarction or atrophy from elevated IOP.
f. Delay of intrinsic retinal vascular development.
g. Accelerated neovascularization or membrane contraction (crunch).
h. Glaucoma or hypotony observed on follow-up examinations up to 20 months after the BEAT-ROP trail.

Systemic Modulation in ROP

Anti-VEGF and laser therapy offer two different treatments. The current focus on anti-VEGF and laser has brought about different interventional paradigms. One is pharmacological, and the other alters geography and is photo destructive. This focus often overlooks an important third strategy for treating ROP, the modulation of systemic parameters.

Systemic modulation includes techniques such as

1. Transfusing liberally,
2. Keeping the O_2 saturation low in the first 6 weeks of life (usually in the 80 to low 90 s to prevent vasoobliteration after 4 h of constriction the architecture never dilates).
3. Avoiding growth factors such as erythropoietin, which is often given to correct anemia but may also stimulate retinal neovascularization.
4. Increasing the O_2 levels to the high 90 s when pre-threshold ROP appears. (usually after 6 weeks) since retinal vessels have auto-regulations, an increase in O_2 makes the plus disease deminish. The findings of the STOP-ROP study did not receive much credit because of the high p value but there was an observed trend where stage three plus disease diminished.

Current Anti-VEGF Treatment Guidelines

Guidelines for anti-VEGF treatment are not universally accepted and current treatment varies from clinician to clinician. The BEAT-ROP study was monitored by the FDA and paved the way for widespread acceptance of Avastin (bevacizumab) for ROP in North America in an off-label manner. However, it is still not agreed when it should be used.

Some countries in Latin America and Asia are giving bevacizumab as universal treatment and have claimed universal success. These countries have had the most experience with Avastin for ROP because they started well before the Americans got approval for use. There are multiple case series with thousands of patients. Some groups that are using it universally claim that recurrences or retinal detachments do not occur. Experience of our group and others throughout the United States strongly suggest that late complications of anti-VEGF therapy occur with regularity, and include the following

1. Smoldering ROP.
2. Late retinal detachment.
3. Late macular dragging.
4. Late epiretinal membrane.
5. Late macular fold.
6. Late neovascularization and vitreous hemorrhage.

There are many who do not believe that anti-VEGF treatment resolves the disease in the same manner that ablative laser does. Ablative laser is akin to 'fixing it and forgetting it'. If you are not able to reliably follow the child, then laser ablation becomes a more favorable option over pharmacological anti-VEGF treatment.

An important consideration in BEAT-ROP is that the study end point was at 57 weeks. Regrettably, this is too early as the timeline of the disease is altered dramatically after injecting anti-VEGF. As a participant of BEAT-ROP we have seen many enrolled cases develop traction or proliferation after the endpoint of data submission. Our group examined patients who had anti-VEGF treatment at or around their first birthday and found that one-third had concerning peripheral retinal vascular phenomenon, including

1. Smoldering fibrovascular proliferation.
2. Wide zones of non-perfusion.

3. Leaking and dilated blind-ending vessels.
4. Late traction formation.

Parents of infants with ROP need to have a basic understanding of the disease process, the possibility of complications, and further interventions. Given the broad range of potential complications from ROP, parents of premature infants need to understand the importance of consistent care and follow-up with a pediatric ophthalmologist who is familiar with ROP and the complications that may arise. Consistency in follow-up appointments is crucial because complications can present at any time [17].

Since avastin therapy may delay vascularization of the peripheral retina, with recurrence can occur more frequently than laser therapy. For this reason why one of the requirements for anti-VEGF monotherapy is commitment by parents to close, long term, follow up. Ideally, this would occur on a biweekly basis until the retinal vessels extend within 2 disk diameters of the ora serrata or the peripheral retina receives late ablation. We prefer to guide later ablative therapy with fluorescein angiography, which clearly delineates the hypo-perfused zones.

The increased burden associated with following these patients coupled with the more frequent clinic visits makes anti-VEGF a more taxing treatment modality, but well worth the effort if peripheral vision loss and myopia can be avoided. Laser treated stage 3+ ROP or AP-ROP eyes have been shown to have significantly higher prevalence of myopia and high myopia when compared with bevacizumab monotherapy in both zones I and II posterior ROP [16]. The value of long-term, regular follow-up of eyes that experience threshold ROP is significant, as new structural findings and retinal detachments are seen in eyes even at 10 years of age.

Experience dictates that children who do not vascularize to the periphery by 75 weeks' post-conception age (typically around the first birthday) require ablation. We usually tell families that if they choose anti-VEGF, they need to commit to a fluorescein angiogram at the first birthday. If the angiogram shows ischemic areas, these are then ablated with laser. We cannot leave preemies with an indefinite state of peripheral non-perfusion.

The addition of anti-VEGF therapy to the armamentarium allows the flexibility to observe rather than treat on some early zone I cases. We can afford to closely observe rather than rush to treat because we have the anti-VEGF available for rapidly advancing cases. The ET-ROP guidelines, while appropriate for the laser era, may not be always appropriate today with the availability of anti-VEGF therapy. Waiting and monitoring if anti-VEGF is required allows for fewer babies to require treatment in early Zone I cases. If ROP resolves spontaneously, the retinal vessels are more likely to develop to the ora serrata than if anti-VEGF therapy was used early; this is the best possible outcome as they do not require any intervention and get well on their own.

Anti-VEGF monotherapy has the benefits of being elegant, specific, and nondestructive; it avoids anterior segment ischemia and iris/lens. It allows preservation of visual field especially in Zone I disease, and there is a reduction in the degree of myopia. Anti-VEGF monotherapy is simple, quick, and can be done under topical anesthetic, without the need for sedation or general anesthesia. Furthermore, the use of Anti-VEGF agents spares the fragile infant from intubation, post-operative steroids, and cycloplegics that each come with their own side effect profiles.

When to Treat with Anti-VEGF

Which cases are most appropriately treated with Bevacizumab? A simple grading system was developed by Dr. Tawansy after retrospective study of 100 cases of AP-ROP and 310 acute ROP detachments. The Vascular Activity Score (VAS) has five different categories, with a maximum score of 10 points. It correlates linearly with anatomic failure after Pars Plana Vitrectomy and helps to guide Avastin therapy.

1. Fetal Vessels.
2. Extent of Plus Disease.
3. Shunt Width.
4. Neovascularization.
5. Hemorrhage or exudate.

A VAS score of >6 would be an indication for primary anti-VEGF therapy.

When to treat with anti-VEGF

1. If the disease is posterior to the equator.
2. If there is a high vascular burden.
3. If there is impending retinal detachment.
4. If part of the retina is detached.
5. If there is vitreous hemorrhage obstructing the view.
6. If the pupil is myotic and will not dilate.
7. If there is any other medio-opacity such as a congenital cataract.
8. If you are planning to do a vitreectomy to clear blood or repair retinal detachment.
9. If the child is too ill to tolerate laser treatment.
10. Planned combination therapy/late detection.
11. In borderline cases if the family is committed to follow-up.

ROP Crunch

ROP Crunch is a phenomena observed in cases where bevacizumab is injected relatively late in the course of ROP. While the drug decreases retinal neovascularization, bevacizumab can also promote progression of the disease to retinal detachment when there is a significant burden of traction on the retina. Bevacizumab and other Anti-VEGF agents have been used for primary therapy, salvage therapy, and for differing degrees of disease such as; threshold disease, type I pre-threshold disease, stage 3 alone, and stage 4a diseases. It is debuted when and how often we need to inject with bevacizumab. Current literature and practical experiences have shown that timing is crucial for success. Late use results in disasterous ROP Crunch. If used too early bevacizumab may cause significant delay of normal retinal vascularization. The former, ROP Crunch, progresses rapidly to inoperable retinal detachment. Evidence has been shown, in cases where conventional laser treatment has failed, that intravitreal bevacizumab is effective as an adjunct to laser or surgery [18]. If the disease progresses after the initial injection, one may; inject additional anti-VEGF or opt to use conventional laser treatment. It is important to note that in these cases it is up to the discretion of the treating surgeon to ascertain which steps to take.

Different Types of Anti-VEGF

Two types of anti-VEGF are available for the treatment of ROP: Avastin (bevacizumab) and Lucentis (ranacizumab). Both have similar clinical effects; their differences are related to molecular size and practicality. A major consideration is the cost difference, which usually favors Avastin. This is important as many health insurance companies currently do not reimburse for the use of anti-VEGF agents in ROP.

Avastin is a bigger molecule, implying that it is more likely to remain within the vitreous cavity instead of escaping into the systemic circulation. Systemic side effects are a concern; premature infants have vascular development occurring throughout their entire bodies. The Anti-VEGF could adversely affect the normal vascularization of developing organs. While there have not been any serious documented side effects, a study has explored the effect of anti-VEGF on brown fat in new born mice. The study demonstrated reduced levels of brown fat following injection with anti-VEGF: "There is a transient, but significant impact of intravitreally administered anti-VEGF antibody on brown adipose tissue in neonatal mice [19].

Vascular activity goes down dramatically within 24 h of Avastin injection in virgin eyes and the effect is sustained (see Figs. 8.7 and 8.8).

However, this treatment is not nearly as effective in salvage therapy of eyes having prior ablation most likely the Anti-VEGF escapes the vitreous cavity through fenestrations neonatal by laser treatment. Once neovascularization resolves and intrinsic vessels cross the ridge (usually within one to two weeks), the growth delay can be variable, making follow-up all the more critical in these patients. Per BEAT-ROP, bevacizumab therapy is associated with fewer recurrences than laser therapy at the study end point. However, when we have followed these eyes over subsequent months, late recurrences have been seen with increased frequency in bevacizumab treated eyes. Recurrences arise at two distinct locations, the leading edge of vascular development and the original fibrovascular ridge/EFP complex. Most vascularize to the ora, while one-third remain non-perfused, leading to smoldering ROP and late dragging or retinal detachment at any time.

When to Treat with Laser

Treatment with Laser is recommended for the following situations:

1. When the disease is typical.
2. When the disease is anterior to equator.
3. When the vascular burden is not great.

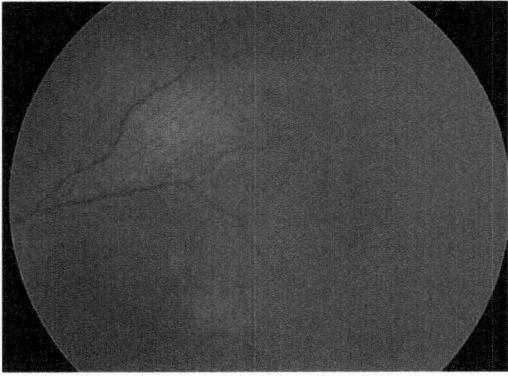

Fig. 8.7 Reduced vascular activity 36 h post anti-VEGF

Fig. 8.8 Reduced vascular activity 36 h post anti-VEGF

4. In cases of smoldering ROP.
5. If the family is unreliable for follow-up or they live at a distance.

Considering Dual Treatment

Should one ever consider both treatments in the same sitting? Yes if the disease is posterior, vascularly active, and there is a good chance the child will be lost to follow up. In dual treatment you can give laser anterior to the equator and anticipate that the intrinsic vasculature will reach the edge of the laser area. When feasible it is preferable to administer Avastin 48 h prior to ablation, thereby preventing its escape through fenestrations caused by the laser. In salvage therapy, serial anti-VEGF injections are required as the drug readily escapes through laser-induced channels. This also significantly increases the risk of systemic toxicity.

Anti-VEGF Dose

A topic of interest arising from the BEAT-ROP study is the dose of anti-VEGF. A 'correct' dose has yet to be worked out systematically. The BEAT-ROP study used a dose of 0.625 mg, half the typical adult dose. This amount was selected on the basis of practical issues without much knowledge of how much anti-VEGF is required. A premature infant's eye cannot tolerate much more than 0.625 mg unless it is concentrated. Importantly, higher doses should be avoided as the increased volume can raise occlude pressure and occlude the central retinal artery. It is crucial to recognize the relationship between volume and radius. The concept of volume being proportional to the radius to the power of 3 means a smaller radial diameter affects the volume much more. Thus, even though these eyes are only one fourth shorter than adults, their volume is one-sixth; this places a constraint on the maximum dose. Additionally, lower doses of bevacizumab may imply less tendency to suppress intrinsic retinal vascular development, thereby lowering the associated risk of Smoldering ROP. A dose response study has yet to been done to assess these issues. Higher doses can be given, and as much as ¾ of the adult dose may be warranted in very severe cases. Reinjection weeks later due to recurrence is sometimes, but rarely, necessary. Clinical response can be seen within 28–48 h in terms of reduction of plus disease in diminishing of the tunica vasculosa lentis, melting away of the ridge, and fading of extra retinal neovascularization. The term 'hell freezes over' is akin to what is seen. Subsequent to the injection, almost nothing happens within the first month and vascular development becomes stagnant. As the anti-VEGF fades, the intrinsic vascular retinal development resumes along with extra retinal neovascularization.

Injection Technique

There are certain considerations to take before injecting anti-VEGF agents. The lens is disproportionately large in preemies, and they do not have a pars plana Traumatic cataract is a catastrophe, as performing cataract surgery in a preterm infant with ROP and ischemia is associated with re-proliferation and pupillary closure. The reason is due to the high rate of re-proliferation and the inability to effectively remove the entire lens (One of the risk factors for proliferative membrane is early lensectomy in a premature child as it is not possible to remove the entire lens. Early lensectomy has a very high incidence of re-proliferation). Avoid hitting the lens at all costs. It is safer to perforate the retina than it is to hit the lens. The BEAT-ROP study demonstrate that a retinal perforation in nonvascularized retina may seal without leadling to retinal detachment.

The injection is given with a sterile technique using betadine prep and cotton pledget with tetracaine or piperacaine to anesthetize the eye. A 31 gauge 5 mm needle is used on an insulin syringe and is primed so that there is no dead space in the needle. The injection is typically given 1 mm posterior to limbus and directed towards the equator rather than towards the posterior pole. Enter temporally and going further temporal to avoid hitting the lens. Always check the optic nerve perfusion and IOP afterwards to ensure good perfusion.

Tips for using laser in type 1 or AP-ROP

1. Study the circulation carefully and try to define the anterior edge of intrinsic vasculature. One can be fooled by flat neovascularization and normal choroidal vessels in posterior cases. Fluorescein angiography is often a helpful guide.
2. Be aware that the amount of laser energy required to get a good take may be significantly higher in the posterior retina than in the periphery. Titrate power appropriately.
3. In a highly vascular eye, be careful not to depress or manipulate the globe with force as it will lead to hemorrhage and leakage from the tunica vasculosa lentis.
4. Consider titrating the amount of laser treatment given and distributing it over several sessions. One might want to titrate it and break it up int. By doing this you can monitor the treatment response and minimize

inflammation and choroidal effusion. It may be easier on the child.
5. Avoid hitting the iris or the tunica vasculosa lentis.
6. Consider light treatment over flat neovascularization and also consider in refractory cases treating directly over the ridge or feeder vessels that perfuse the ridge.
7. Avoid treating retina that is detached as it can create holes; cryo can be used for these areas.
8. Consider using cryo in areas of robust neovascularization.
9. When doing serial laser treatments, consider using minimally invasive anesthesia such as oral sucrose and acetaminophen rather than intubation.

Beware of flat neovascularization. Do not confuse this with the edge of vascular development. The edge of the normal vessels may be further posterior if there exists flat neovascularization. Areas of flat neovascularization that are covering the retina need to be treated but care must be taken as they tend to bleed. When treating posterior disease, the power requirements are often higher. It may be reasonable to break the laser treatment up into multiple sittings. Avoid putting in too much energy at once because it will cause choroidal effusion and a higher chance of anterior segment ischemia. Avoid treating the long posterior ciliary neurovascular bundle that travels within the choroid at 3 and 9 o'clock positions; ablation of these can create anterior segment ischemia and lead to corneal opacity, cataract, and massive fibrin production. Sometimes retinopathy can be controlled by treating the neovascularization itself and 'strangulating' it by getting to the base of its blood supply. Generally, we think it is potentially dangerous to put in more than 500 spots in any given session. Be gentle about manipulating eyes with posterior disease because they often have an active tunica vasculosa lentis which are the fetal vessels.

Conclusion

The rising prevalence of ROP throughout the world in association with modernization of neonatal intensive care units remains a major health concern. There have been significant advances in the treatment of AP-ROP since the fundamental findings of the CRYO-ROP study. Retinal vascular development, plus disease, retinal neovascularization, and apoptosis of fetal vessels can be manipulated by systemic variables such as oxygen saturation, nutrition, and hemoglobin levels. In conjunction with systemic manipulation, proven local therapies such as retinal ablation with laser or cryotherapy, anti-VEGF agents, and possibly steroids are currently the standard of care. With different approaches to treatment, management strategies and treatment paradigms vary amongst centers and differ widely. Present-day treatment is more like a chess match rather than a cook book recipe. In prior years, ophthalmologists followed the CRYO-ROP recommendation of 5 contiguous or 8 cumulative clock hours, and the decision of whether to laser was based on the presence of threshold. Later, some started treating pre-threshold and ET-ROP validated this notion. STOP-ROP reduced the progression from pre-threshold to threshold in certain cases with maintenance of high oxygen saturation. Laser treatment has evolved into several techniques, including confluent, semi confluent, near confluent, serial, into the ridge, or over flat neovascularization. It can be directed focally into areas of ischemia or cover the entire avascular retina.

The introduction of anti-VEGF agents brought questions responding the different types of anti-VEGF, dosages, timing of administration, and serial versus single injections. In combination therapy utilizing two or more modalities, the order of each treatment used is another variable to consider. The vascular activity score can help guide the decision making process. The experience of the treating surgeon should also be taken into account as treatment is dependent upon, level of comfort, in using specific therapies. With new ideas and proven therapies being used together, currently there exists no uniform protocol in the treatment of ROP.

It is important to remember that anti-VEGF is not a panacea; treatment requires committed follow-up and may eventually necessitate late laser ablation. Laser remains the most proven in terms of 'putting the disease to bed', so if we only had one choice it would be laser. It is helpful to follow the above listed practical techniques and methodologies when using laser, anti-VEGF, or dual therapy. Collected data from the landmark studies and practical clinical experiences myriad an approach to the different circumstances and characteristics that are encountered with ROP. The myriad of approaches, techniques, and treatments need to be orchestrated synergistically, considering modalities in conjunction as well as in single application. The overarching goal is to be as minimally invasive as possible while achieving excellent visual outcomes for all babies.

References

1. Chen J, Smith LEH. Retinopathy of prematurity. Angiogenesis. 2007;10.2:133–40 (Web).
2. Chen J, Stahl A, Hellstrom A, Smith LE. Current update on retinopathy of prematurity: screening and treatment. Curr Opin Pediatr. 2011;23(2):173–8.
3. Leung DW, Cachianes G, Kuang WJ, Goeddel DV, Ferrara N. Vascular endothelial growth factor is a secreted angiogenic mitogen. Science. 1989;246:1306–9.
4. Senger DR, Galli SJ, Dvorak AM, Perruzzi CA, Harvey VS, Dvorak HF. Tumor cells secrete a vascular permeability factor that promotes accumulation of ascites fluid. Science. 1983;219:983–5.
5. Adamis AP, Shima DT, Yeo KT, Yeo TK, Brown LF, Berse B, D'Amore PA, Folkman J. Synthesis and secretion of vascular permeability factor/vascular endothelial growth factor by human retinal pigment epithelial cells. Biochem Biophys Res Commun. 1993;193:631–8.
6. Chan-Ling T, Gock B, Stone J. The effect of oxygen on vasoformative cell division. Evidence that 'physiological hypoxia' is the stimulus for normal retinal vasculogenesis. Invest Ophthalmol Vis Sci. 1995;36:1201–14.
7. Patz A. Clinical and experimental studies on retinal neovascularization. XXXIX Edward Jackson memorial lecture. Am J Ophthalmol. 1982;94:715–43.

8. Roth AM. Retinal vascular development in premature infants. Am J Ophthalmol. 1977;84.5:636–40 (Web).

9. Donahue ML, Phelps DL, Watkins RH, Lomonaco MB, Horowitz S. Retinal vascular endothelial growth factor (VEGF) MRNA expression is altered in relation to neovascularization in oxygen induced retinopathy. Curr Eye Res. 1996;15.2:175–84 (Web).

10. Young TL, Anthony DC, Pierce E, Foley E, Smith LE. Histopathology and vascular endothelial growth factor in untreated and diode laser-treated retinopathy of prematurity. J Am Assoc Pediatr Ophthalmol Strabismus. 1997;1.2:105–10 (Web).

11. Good WV. Final results of the early treatment for retinopathy of prematurity (ETROP) randomized trial. Trans Am Ophthalmol Soc. 2004;102:233–250 (on behalf of the early treatment for retinopathy of prematurity cooperative group).

12. Tah V, Orlans HO, Hyer J, et al. Anti-VEGF therapy and the retina: an update. J Ophthalmol. 2015;Article ID 627674:13. doi:10.1155/2015/627674.

13. Gole GA, Elis AL, Katz X, Holmstrom G, Fielder AR, Capone A Jr, Flynn JT, Good WG, Holmes JM, McNamara A, Palmer EA, Quinn GE, Shapiro MJ, Trese MGJ, Wallace DK. The international classification of retinopathy of prematurity revisited. Arch Ophthalmol Arch Ophthalmol. 2005;123.7:991–99 (Web).

14. Palmer EA, Hardy RJ, Dobson V, Phelps DL, Quinn GE, Summers CG, Krom CP, Tung B. Cryotherapy of retinopathy of prematurity cooperative group. 15-year outcomes following threshold retinopathy of prematurity. Arch Ophthalmol Arch Ophthalmol. 2005;123.3:311 (Web. Payment coming).

15. Dobson V, Quinn GE, Summers CG, Hardy RJ, Tung B, Good WV. Grating visual acuity results in the early treatment for retinopathy of prematurity study. Arch Ophthalmol. 2011;129(7):840–6 (Early Treatment for retinopathy of prematurity cooperative group).

16. Mintz-Hittner HA, Kennedy KA, Chuang AZ. BEAT-ROP cooperative group. Efficacy of intravitreal bevacizumab for stage 3+ retinopathy of prematurity. N Engl J Med. 2011;364(7):603–615 (1000$ Payment coming).

17. Kuerschner DR. Does my child really need to wear these glasses? A review of retinopathy of prematurity and long-term outcomes. 2003. http://www.medscape.com/viewarticle/461578. (N.p., Web).

18. Geloneck MM, Chuang AZ, Clark WL, Hunt MG, Norman AA, Packwood EA, Tawansy KA, Mintz-Hittner HA. Refractive outcomes following bevacizumab monotherapy compared with conventional laser treatment. JAMA Ophthalmol JAMA Ophthalmol. 2014;132.11:1327–1333 (Web).

19. Jo DH, SW Park, Cho CS, Powner MB, Kim JH, Fruttiger M, Kim JH. Intravitreally injected Anti-VEGF antibody reduces brown fat in neonatal mice. PLOS ONE. 2015;10.7 (n. pag. Web).

Management of Stage 4 ROP

Andrés Kychenthal B. and Paola Dorta S.

Abstract

Successfully managing stage 4A ROP retinal detachment, that is, a partial detachment not involving the fovea, is the last opportunity of obtaining good vision in these eyes. The onset of stage 4 is thus a therapeutic window that cannot be missed. All efforts must be placed on a timely diagnosis and intervention. Performing a lens-sparing vitrectomy in eyes with stage 4 ROP results in very good anatomical and functional outcomes in the majority of the cases. The use of antiVEGF drugs prior to the vitreoretinal surgery, to induce regression of the neovascular activity, can further improve these results and allow earlier and safer interventions.

Keywords

Retinopathy of prematurity (ROP) · Retinal detachment · Neovascular activity · Vitrectomy · Bevacizumab

Introduction

Despite efforts for adequate screening and treatment, retinal detachment does continue to occur in some patients with ROP. Although retinal ablation is effective in most cases of threshold ROP, 12% of the eyes in the early treatment for retinopathy of prematurity (ETROP) randomized trial detached before 9 months corrected age despite timely peripheral ablation [1]. Advanced ROP remains a significant problem in many countries around the world, being the leading cause of childhood blindness in many of them. ROP has been affecting emerging economies and middle-income countries where the rates of disease requiring treatment tend to be higher [2, 3].

An increase in the more posterior forms of the disease and the lack of a timely diagnosis or treatment are responsible for the occurrence of some of these cases.

Although the introduction of anti-proliferative therapy might improve outcomes and thus decrease the occurrence of retinal detachments, there are very important issues associated with the

Andrés Kychenthal B. (✉) · Paola Dorta S.
Ophthalmology, KYDOFT Foundation, Av Luis
Pasteur 5280 of 304, Santiago, Chile
e-mail: akychenthal@kydoft.cl

use of these drugs in relation to retinal detachments. First, for the drug to be effective it has to be injected at the appropriate time. There are still too many places where ROP screening is not good enough and a timely intervention will not be possible. If the antiVEGF is injected too late, it might provoke or accelerate the development of a retinal detachment. Second, late onset detachments can occur in babies treated with these drugs even many weeks after an initial regression.

Visual outcome in eyes with retinopathy of prematurity-related retinal detachment is generally very poor [4, 5]. Neither the stability of the detachment nor the progression rate is predictable following peripheral retinal ablation or after the use of antiVEGF drugs [6, 7]. On the other hand, adequate treatment can achieve good anatomical and functional results [8–15].

The purpose when treating these cases is to obtain as much vision as possible. When the macula is still attached, the anatomical success rate is approximately 90% [10–12, 15] and the goal is an undistorted or minimally distorted posterior pole, total retinal reattachment with preservation of the lens and visual acuity in the range of 20/60 [9, 14].

Surgical options for the management of stage 4 ROP include vitrectomy, either lens sparing or combined vitrectomy lensectomy, and scleral buckle.

This chapter will focus on the management of stage 4A ROP, that is, macula-sparing detachments. When a partial detachment is present but the macula is involved (Stage 4B), the anatomical and visual objectives are more closely related to cases with a total retinal detachment or stage 5.

There are many elements that are essential to ROP surgery, the keys to a successful outcome being when and how these cases should be treated.

General Considerations

Surgical Team

A surgeon willing to address ROP retinal detachments should keep in mind that pediatric

and especially ROP surgery is substantially different from vitreoretinal interventions performed in adults. Proper training is thus required.

To do a safe operation on these very sick preterms, the surgical team should include a skilled pediatric anesthesiologist and a whole group of professionals beyond the operating room. The surgical intervention is only one element in the objective of achieving not only good anatomical but also good functional results. Refractive treatments and managing amblyopia also play a significant part. Pediatric ophthalmologists, neonatologists, vision therapists, and support staff all play a role in the management of these patients.

Surgical Anatomy

It must be taken into consideration by the surgeon that he will be operating on a small eye, that preterms infants do not have a developed pars plana [16] and that the lens is proportionally bigger than in the fully developed eye. Entry sites when performing a lens-sparing vitrectomy should be only 0.5 mm posterior to the limbus [17]. In those eyes that have been previously photocoagulated, this distance might be increased to 1–1.5 mm, thus minimizing the threat to the lens [18]. It is worth noting that the lens will not become cataractous, if it is only touched by the instruments and the lens capsule remains intact. If the surgical plan is to remove the lens, then entering through the limbus would be adequate in order to avoid any chance of inadvertent retinal damage.

These particular anatomical issues should be added to the particular configuration of the detachment in order to define the most appropriate surgical approach for each case.

It should always be taken into consideration that neither pre- nor postoperative retinal anatomy is predictive of the visual potential of an eye. There are eyes that although having very distorted retinas have better than 20/40 vision, and on the other hand some eyes that have very good anatomical results might see very poorly [19].

Preoperative Examination

In most cases, the retinal status of a preterm patient can be determined in the neonatal intensive care unit or in the office, but it is recommended to perform a complete ocular assessment as the first step in all surgical cases to confirm the configuration and the extent of the detachment, determine the best surgical plan including entry sites and also to take images of the retinal status. Sometimes this examination can be performed under anesthesia just prior to the surgical intervention. A good preoperative record of the retinal status will serve both follow-up and medico-legal purposes.

Informed Consent

A detailed informed consent should be signed by the parents or legal guardian of the child. In addition to the potential benefits and risk of the procedure, it is advisable to state that the visual potential of an eye might be affected by many factors, not only ocular but also systemic and developmental. Thus, no certainty regarding the amount of vision can be promised at that point.

Postoperative Care and Follow-up

Postoperative posturing can be very difficult to achieve in cases where face down positioning is required. Parents can help in this task at least for 1 or 2 days. Preventing the child from removing the eye patch or rubbing the eye can also be a challenging task for the supporting staff.

Evaluation of the retinal status can also be difficult in the immediate postoperative period. Measuring the eye's pressure can be very difficult if not impossible and thus efforts to prevent postoperative hypotony or glaucoma should be taken into account in the surgical technique. Although suturing all sclerotomies is mandatory when using 20 gauge instruments to prevent

hypotony, sutureless techniques with 25 gauge systems have proven to be safe [15].

In the follow-up of these patients, examination under anesthesia will sometimes be the only way to perform a complete assessment.

Timing of the Surgery

The timing in which the surgery for a ROP-related retinal detachment is performed is one of the key elements to obtaining good results. It always has to be taken into consideration by everybody involved in the management of these cases that:

- The time frame for an effective treatment is short.
- The more advanced the detachment the worse the anatomic and functional results.
- The stability of detachments is unpredictable and their progression rate is variable. Even partial retinal detachments can be associated with extremely poor vision if left untreated.

There had been a misunderstanding that stage 4A might be stable and surgery should be performed only after the macula is detached. Data from the Cryo-ROP study showed that partial detachments present three months after threshold ROP are unstable anatomically, and the visual outcome is generally poor. The best predictor of structural outcome was the total area of the detached retina as measured by the number of segments of detached retina from the total of 34 segments: 92% of the eyes with 13 or more segments had unfavorable structural outcome.

If retinal detachment occurs, the best chance for a favorable outcome occurs when the detachment does not progress beyond three segments [5] (Fig. 9.1).

This means that fixing initial detachments is the last opportunity of preserving good vision in these babies and that makes stage 4A a therapeutic window that cannot be missed.

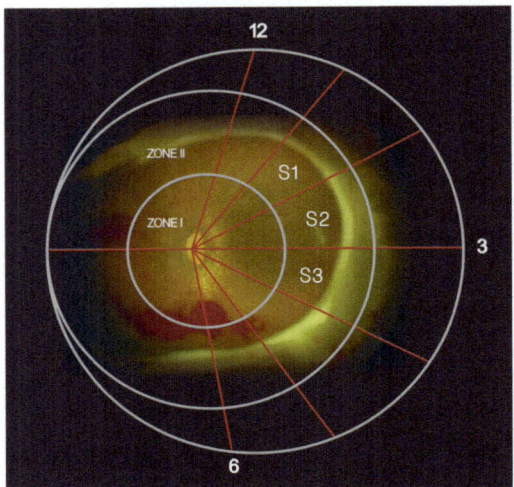

Fig. 9.1 Schematic representation of zones and segments of ROP classification superimposed on a clinical image of a stage 4A detachment. If retinal detachment develops, the best chance for a favorable outcome occurs when the detachment does not progress beyond 3 of the 34 segments

In eyes that were treated by laser prior to the development of the detachment, surgical intervention has typically been performed at approximately 40 weeks postconceptional age, classically between 38 and 42 weeks.

If adequate follow-up of the case is possible, adjustments within this range and to this general rule are induced mainly by the presence of active vascularity. The presence of active vascular activity is a serious problem leading to unfavorable surgical results, and thus many authors advocate waiting before performing vitreous surgery until they find a vascularly quiet eye [9, 10, 20, 21]. The use of antiVEGF drugs in recent years has prompted changes in this timing, shifting interventions to earlier postconceptional ages.

In cases of aggressive posterior ROP (AP-ROP), some authors have advocated very early surgical intervention, even performing a vitrectomy before the presence of a retinal detachment [22]. Now it seems more appropriate to first use antiVEGF drugs, which have proved very effective in these very severe cases of ROP [23–28].

Great success rates can be achieved when operating on stage 4A ROP. All efforts should be made not to wait, but to intervene as soon as possible when this diagnosis is made.

Surgical Techniques

General Aspects

As essential as the timing, that is when an operation on ROP patients with retinal detachment should be performed, is how that surgical intervention is carried out. The surgical technique is thus a main element in achieving good results.

There is more than one surgical option to treat a stage 4 retinal detachment. These options include mainly scleral buckling, lens-sparing vitrectomy, and combined lensectomy–vitrectomy. These procedures in turn can be performed with diverse surgical techniques. The use of pharmacological aids might also play a significant role in the management of these detachments, and their use must therefore be taken into consideration.

Each case should be evaluated independently, and all local and systemic factors should be included in the deliberation to decide the best surgical approach for each eye.

The goal in surgical procedures for stage 4 ROP is mainly to stop the shrinkage and traction of the fibrotic tissue developed from the regression of the neovascularization. As previously mentioned, both vitrectomy and scleral buckle can be used to treat stage 4. Considering that vitreous surgery can effectively interrupt the progression of ROP retinal detachment by directly addressing trans-vitreal traction resulting from fibrous proliferation and that when preserving the lens there is much less risk of amblyopia and better chances of central fixation with better vision, lens-sparing vitrectomy is our preferred surgical approach.

Scleral Buckling

Scleral buckling can be effective for treating ROP-related retinal detachments. Different anatomical results and reattachment rates have been published for stages 4A, 4B and 5 [29–32]. With current surgical techniques and instrumentation, vitreoretinal surgery seems a more direct and effective method of addressing trans-vitreal traction. Better results have been reported with vitrectomy for stage 4 when compared to scleral buckling [33]. Adding a scleral buckle does not increase the success of lens-sparing vitreoretinal interventions in stage 4 [34].

Notwithstanding, a scleral buckle can be considered for some cases, particularly when traction is mainly located anterior to the equator. It has also been used in the more effusive types of detachment [35]. These more effusive detachments can sometimes be observed in the acute phase of the disease or following cryotherapy.

Scleral Buckle Technique (Encircling Band)

Like the majority of the authors, we favor the use of an encircling scleral buckle (Figs. 9.2, 9.3), although others have reported successful outcomes using segmental scleral buckling [32].

The technique of scleral buckling in our ROP patients involves:

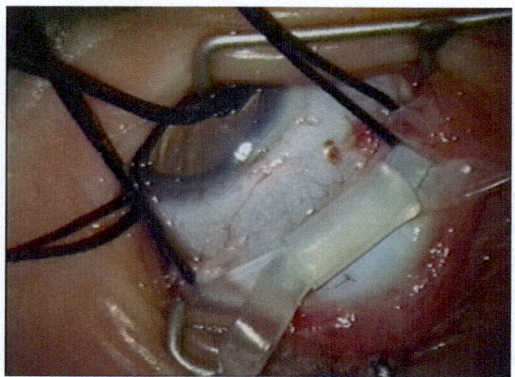

Fig. 9.2 Image of a scleral buckle, a 2.5 mm solid silicone band. A good scleral indentation can be observed

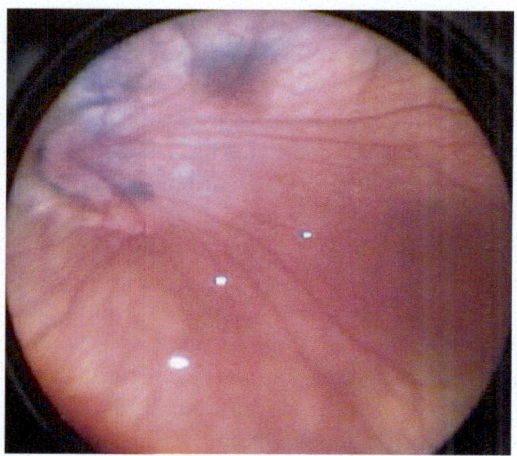

Fig. 9.3 Picture of the posterior pole of a case with stage 4A in a Zone I ROP treated with a scleral buckle taken one year after surgery. Despite distortion of the macular area a 20/60 vision was observed at the age of 14 years in this patient

- 360° peritomy at the limbus, isolation of the four rectus muscles follow by a silk suture passed under each of them for handling.
- A cotton tip is used to strip the sclera in all four quadrants.
- A 2.5 mm # 240 solid silicone band is sutured to the sclera using 5-0 non-reabsorbable sutures. The band is placed at the equator and supporting the ridge when possible.
- Proper tightening is done by performing a paracentesis with a 30 gauge needle mounted in a tuberculin syringe to drain aqueous fluid. The perfusion status of the central artery should be checked after the final tightening of the band.

Although the anatomical success rate of buckling procedures can be fairly good, the functional results are much worse. Encircling buckles induce myopic refractive changes that can be very high and thus potentially amblyogenic. Additionally, possible negative effects of the encircling band on choroidal circulation should be considered. The eye grows significantly during the first year so a moderate buckling effect at the time of surgery can lead to much greater constriction over time. To address this problem, division or removal of the band is recommended when stable retinal reattachment is achieved. [36]. This is usually done after 6 months if retinal reattachment is stable or in cases of anisometropia, however it seems logical to delay the removal in unstable situations. A two-step intervention with elongation of the buckle has also been proposed to allow an almost constant buckling effect during the first year of life [37].

Concerns regarding amblyopia with scleral buckling, improvements in surgical techniques and instrumentation, the very infrequent use of cryotherapy leading to effusive cases and the availability of antiVEGF drugs as adjuncts for intraocular surgery have placed buckling as a second choice as opposed to vitrectomy for stage 4 ROP.

It must be emphasized that reattachment of the retina after a buckling procedure for ROP is a slow process that can take several weeks to settle.

Vitrectomy

There are different technical approaches to performing vitreoretinal surgery for retinal detachments in ROP. The surgery can be done using two or three ports and be either standard 20 gauge or micro-incisional vitrectomy surgery. There might not be a preferred technique and at the end it is mostly surgeon-dependent. Each surgeon should use the technique that produces the best possible results in his/her hands.

A careful preoperative examination will allow the best entry site to the vitreous cavity to be chosen. An open space between the retina and the lens is necessary to perform a lens-sparing vitrectomy. If there is advanced anterior retinal traction there is a high risk of causing a retinal break, and an anterior approach should be selected.

Lens-Sparing Vitrectomy (LSV)

Surgical technique to perform LSV using a 3-port, 25-gauge trans-conjunctival sutureless approach:

- Sclerotomies are made 0.5–1.0 mm posterior to the limbus through the pars plicata. In the first place, the conjunctiva is displaced immediately above the sclerotomy site and the cannula is inserted into the vitreous cavity using a beveled trocar. This procedure is applied to place the cannulas in the temporal, superotemporal, and superonasal quadrants. The infusion cannula is placed in the temporal quadrant while the superotemporal and superonasal ports are used to pass the light pipe and the cutter.

- Vitrectomy and membrane peeling are performed with settings of >1500 cpm and a suction of 500 mmHg. The cutter must be used very cautiously to avoid any iatrogenic breaks. If a rhegmatogenous component is added during surgery, the chances for a successful outcome are dramatically reduced.

- The aim of the vitrectomy is to dissect the tractional proliferation between the ridge and the lens, the ridge and the nerve, the ridge and the vitreous base, and the circumferential traction along the ridge.

- A partial fluid-air exchange is performed at the end of the procedure in the majority of cases. When fluid is left in the vitreous cavity, the infusion cannula is removed at the last step to check for the need for further infusion.

- The conjunctiva is closed using a bipolar diathermy.

Lensectomy–Vitrectomy

Lensectomy–vitrectomy will be performed in a stage 4 ROP when anterior traction does not make lens sparing a safe choice. Although LSV is the preferred method, it always has to be clear that it is better to remove the lens than to make an entry site break. When the lens is removed, good visual acuity is much less likely. Amblyopia is in most cases severe and difficult to treat. Nonetheless it is important to consider that after a vitrectomy for stage 4 ROP, continuing improvement of vision development can occur over long periods of time. Restoration of the retinal architecture and the plasticity of the infant's developing brain are thought to play a role [38].

The entry site for lensectomy–vitrectomy surgery will be the limbus, just above the plane of the iris root. This will allow for safe removal of the lens and intravitreal maneuvers. Twenty three-gauge instrumentation can be successfully used in pediatric conditions [39, 40], and it might be a good selection of instruments for these cases. Entry sites should be sutured with 10-0 nylon at the end of the procedure.

The small gauge instrumentation currently available allows for effective and safe vitreo-retinal procedures (Fig. 9.4). Initial problems such as instrument flexibility and adequate illumination have been resolved. The use of a specific gauge or a combination of different instrumentation should be available to allow the surgeon to choose the best alternative for each particular case.

Complications of Vitreous Surgery

Hemorrhage: Intra- and postoperative bleeding greatly increases the risk of failure of any intraocular surgical procedure in ROP-related retinal detachments. Eyes that have not had peripheral ablation and that have perfused fibrovascular tissue at the time of surgery are at the highest risk of bleeding. Waiting for spontaneous regression of the neovascular activity was done prior to the availability of antiVEGF drugs.

Hypotony: This can occur during a vitrectomy, and it should be prevented by the use of adequate instrumentation. Avoiding hypotony when using a two-port approach can be challenging and requires great experience. The use of a third port can help to maintain more stable intraoperative pressure. Although trans-conjunctival sutureless vitrectomies using small gauge instrumentation works very well, if there is doubt regarding leakage from any of the entry sites, then a suture should be place to secure the eye closure. The closure of the conjunctiva with a bipolar diathermy in all sutureless cases might also help to prevent hypotony. When the entry sites are through the limbus they should always be sutured.

Retinal breaks: ROP surgery poses a very significant challenge to the surgeon. It is well known that the chances of anatomical success are very small if there is a rhegmatogenous component added to the detachment. If a break is formed during a vitrectomy, the complete release of the traction associated with the break is needed for the surgery to have any chances of success. Special attention must be paid not to induce an entry site break when an anterior proliferation is present.

Endophthalmitis: This is a potential risk in any intraocular intervention. Using all the

(a) (b)

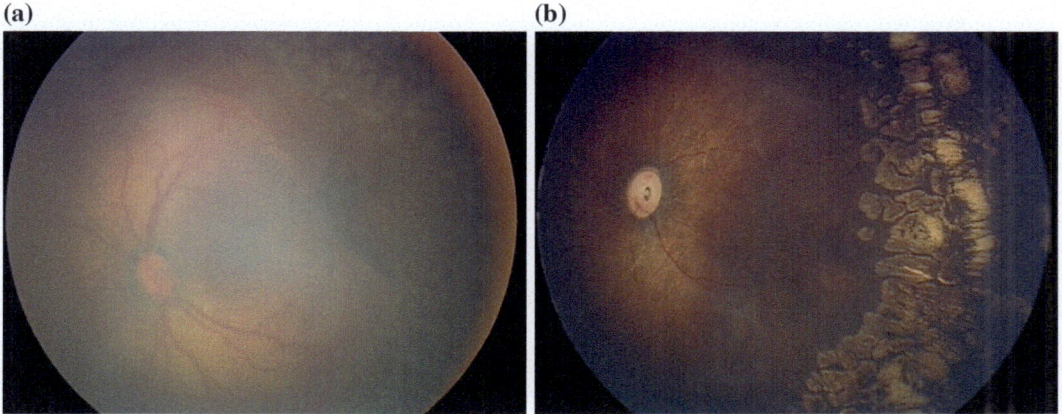

Fig. 9.4 Pre (**a**) and postoperative (**b**) images of the left eye of a preterm born at 29 weeks and 1.200 g that developed a stage 4A retinal detachment that was managed with a vitrectomy performed with 25 gauge instrumentation

standard preoperative measures, suturing limbal entries and closing the conjunctiva with bipolar diathermy in cases of a sutureless approach should prevent it.

Glaucoma: Pressure elevation can occur in the immediate postoperative period, but adequate surgical techniques should make this problem infrequent. Postoperative glaucoma could be a late complication after ROP retinal detachment surgery. [41] Follow-up that includes measurement of the intraocular pressure should be performed in these children.

AntiVEGF Drugs in the Management of Rop Retinal Detachments

The use of antiVEGF drugs in ROP has prompted changes in the management of ROP-related retinal detachments. These drugs might help in the management of patients who already have a detached retina, but they have also created a new category of retinal detachments, those that can develop after using anti-angiogenic agents to treat the acute stages of the disease.

AntiVEGF Drugs as an Adjunct

The presence of vascular activity is a major problem when operating on a ROP retinal detachment. The risk of uncontrollable bleeding and failure of the surgical procedure are much greater in eyes with active vascularity.

AntiVEGF drugs that can be injected prior to the surgical intervention address this issue by inducing rapid regression of vascular activity, allowing one to operate on a vascularly inactive or "quiet eye" rather than on an active one (Fig. 9.5).

Especially significant is the fact that this effect allows the surgery to be carried out without the drawback of a long wait for natural regression of the neovascular activity. Thus, intervention that is earlier than previously possible should prevent progression and macular involvement, offering better visual potential for these eyes [21, 42].

The right time to inject an antiVEGF drug and perform the vitrectomy seems especially important when a retinal detachment is already present. A balance between the neovascular regression and avoiding the development of fibrous tissue with traction on the retina are essential. One week after injecting the antiVEGF drug seems to be a good moment to perform the surgery. In that period of time, a very significant reduction in the vascular activity occurs, allowing for a safe procedure. A longer interval between the injection and the surgery might provoke progression in the detachment or even a rhegmatogenous factor due to traction on the retina induced by the regression and fibrous conversion of the neovascular tissues.

It is worth noting that regression of initial cases of detachment has been observed with the use of antiVEGF drugs alone [21].

Combining the use of antiVEGF drugs with a lens-sparing vitrectomy in stage 4A should give the best results. This approach would add all the benefits of a LSV to being carried out at a very

(a)   (b)   (c)

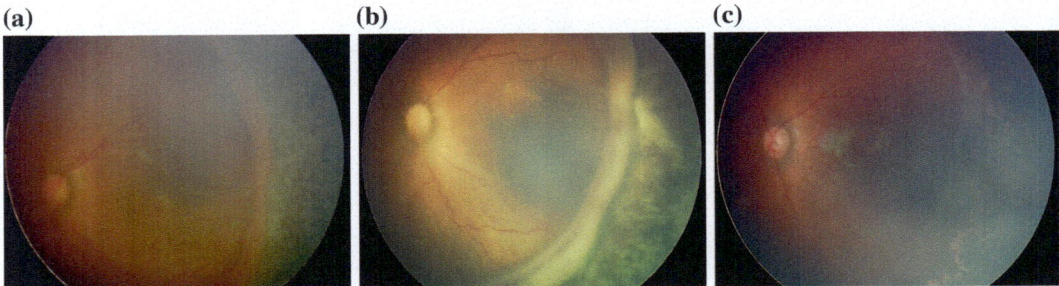

Fig. 9.5 a Stage 4A retinal detachment present at 37 weeks of gestational age in a preterm born at 24 weeks with 760 grams. Due to the significant vascular activity present an antiVEGF drug was injected prior to surgery

b One week after the antiVEGF injection, a marked reduction in the vascular activity could be observed. A 25-gauge lens-sparing vitrectomy was performed at that time. **c** Favorable anatomical outcome 9 weeks after surgery

early stage. As the average time for intervention in 4A detachments has been close to 40 weeks of postconceptional age, this two-step method might allow for operations closer to 38 weeks or even earlier. Retinal vascularization continues growing toward the periphery in what appears to be a normal pattern after treatment with anti-VEGF drugs followed by LSV. The vessels clearly pass the location of the previous detachment and ridge.

Notwithstanding very reasonable safety concerns for the use of these types of drugs in developing babies, the beneficial effect of using such drugs as adjuvants in the treatment of vascularly active retinal detachment cases is immense. The best antiVEGF drug and dose for this purpose are still under investigation.

Additional Pharmacological Surgical Adjuncts

Intravitreal corticosteroids: Triamcinolone has been used to aid in vitreoretinal procedures in ROP-related retinal detachments to address the vascularity problem [43, 44]. Anti-angiogenic drugs as previously discussed are a better choice to address this issue.

Plasmin: The very strong vitreoretinal adhesion in the pediatric population prevents the induction of a posterior vitreous separation during vitrectomy in these patients. The use of autologous plasmin has proven useful in the pediatric population and ROP-related detachments [45–47]. Now microplasmin, a recombinant form of human plasmin, is being studied as a surgical adjunct for pediatric retinal surgery [48]. The potential benefits of such a drug are numerous.

Retinal Detachment After Using AntiVEGF Drugs to Treat Type 1 ROP

Retinal detachments that follow the use of anti-angiogenic drugs can be divided into two different groups.

In the first group, the detachment develops shortly after the injection. A change from vascular to fibrous tissue resulting in traction that pulls on the retina causes the detachment [49]. This could be the result of the progression of the disease or a situation resulting from the use of the antiVEGF drug too late, the so-called "**ROP Crunch.**"

A timely diagnosis and intervention are crucial for a favorable outcome. As with laser treatment, these injections must be performed at the appropriate moment to avoid progression to a retinal detachment.

The second group is composed of patients with a **delayed-onset retinal detachment** despite early regression of the disease after the use of an antiVEGF drug. Some of these cases are especially difficult to diagnose because they can occur many weeks after the injection, when patients are not being appropriately followed up. There are reports of cases even after 60 weeks postconceptional age [7].

Patterns of regression and recurrence are not yet well known in patients treated with anti-angiogenic drugs. The risk of a late onset retinal detachment makes extended follow-up after using antiVEGF injections mandatory. To significantly decrease the chances of a retinal detachment after the use of antiVEGF drugs, either when follow-up over extended periods is not possible or even as a primary approach, laser photocoagulation can be applied to the peripheral retina once these drugs have allowed retinal vasculature to pass zone II.

References

1. Early Treatment for Retinopathy of Prematurity Cooperative Group. Revised indications for the treatment of retinopathy of prematurity: results of the early treatment for retinopathy of prematurity randomized trial. Arch Ophthalmol.
2. Steinkuller PG, Du L, Gilbert C, et al. Childhood blindness. J AAPOS. 1999;3:26–32.
3. Gilbert C. Retinopathy of prematurity: a global perspective of the epidemics, population of babies at risk and implications for control. Early Hum Dev. 2008;84(2):77–82.
4. Cryotherapy for Retinopathy of Prematurity Cooperative Group. Multicenter trial of cryotherapy for retinopathy of prematurity: ophthalmological outcomes at 10 years. Arch Ophthalmol. 2001;119:1110–8.

5. Gilbert W, Quinn GE, Dobson V, et al. Partial retinal detachment at 3 months after threshold retinopathy of prematurity. Long-term structural and functional outcome. Arch Ophthalmol. 1996;114:1085–91.

6. Cryotherapy for Retinopathy of Prematurity Cooperative Group. Multicenter trial of cryotherapy for retinopathy of prematurity: 31/2-year outcome-structure and function. Arch Ophthalmol 1993;111:339–344.

7. Hu J, Blair MP, Shapiro MJ, Lichtenstein SJ, Galasso JM, Kapur R. Reactivation of retinopathy of prematurity after bevacizumab injection. Arch Ophthalmol. 2012;130(8):1000–6. Erratum in: Arch Ophthalmol. 2013;131(2):212.

8. Recchia FM, Capone A Jr. Contemporary understanding and management of retinopathy of prematurity. Retina. 2004;24(2):283–92.

9. Prenner JL, Capone A Jr, Trese MT. Visual outcomes after lens-sparing vitrectomy for stage 4A retinopathy of prematurity. Ophthalmology. 2004;111(12):2271–3.

10. Capone A Jr, Trese MT. Lens-sparing vitreous surgery for tractional stage 4A retinopathy of prematurity retinal detachments. Ophthalmology. 2001;108(11):2068–70.

11. Hubbard GB 3rd, Cherwick DH, Burian G. Lens-sparing vitrectomy for stage 4 retinopathy of prematurity. Ophthalmology. 2004;111(12):2274–7.

12. Moshfeghi AA, Banach MJ, Salam GA, Ferrone PJ. Lens-sparing vitrectomy for progressive tractional retinal detachments associated with stage 4A retinopathy of prematurity. Arch Ophthalmol. 2004;122(12):1816–8.

13. Lakhanpal R, Sun R, Albini T, Holz E. Anatomic success rate after 3-port lens-sparing vitrectomy in stage 4A or 4B retinopathy of prematurity. Ophthalmology. 2005;112:1569–73.

14. Lakhanpal RR, Sun RL, Albini TA, Coffee R, Coats DK, Holz ER. Visual outcomes after 3-port lens-sparing vitrectomy in stage 4 retinopathy of prematurity. Arch Ophthalmol. 2006;124(5):675–9.

15. Kychenthal A, Dorta P. 25-gauge lens-sparing vitrectomy for stage 4A retinopathy of prematurity. Retina. 2008;28(3 Suppl):S65–8.

16. Hairston RJ, Maguire AM, Vitale S, Green WR. Morphometric analysis of pars plana development in humans. Invest Ophthalmol Vis Sci. 1992;33:1197.

17. Lemley Craig A, Han Dennis P. An age-based method for planning sclerotomy placement during pediatric vitrectomy: a 12-year experience. Retina. 2007;27(7):974–7.

18. Capone A. Lens-sparing vitrectomy for posterior retinopathy of prematurity: indications and techniques. Vitreoretinal Surg Technol. 1993;5:3–4.

19. Ferrone PJ, Trese MT, Williams GA, Cox MS. Good visual acuity in an adult population with marked posterior segment changes secondary to retinopathy of prematurity. Retina. 1998;18(4):335–8.

20. Fuchino Y, Hayashi H, Kono T, Ohshima K. Long term follow-up of visual acuity in eyes with stage 5 retinopathy of prematurity after closed vitrectomy. Am J Ophthalmol. 1995;120:308–16.

21. Kychenthal A, Dorta P. Vitrectomy after intravitreal bevacizumab (Avastin) for retinal detachment in retinopathy of prematurity. Retina. 2010;30(4 Suppl):S32–6.

22. Azuma N(1), Ishikawa K, Hama Y, Hiraoka M, Suzuki Y, Nishina S. Early vitreous surgery for aggressive posterior retinopathy of prematurity. Am J Ophthalmol. 2006;142(4):636–43.

23. Mintz-Hittner Helen A, Kennedy Kathleen A, Chuang Alice Z. Efficacy of intravitreal bevacizumab for stage 3 + retinopathy of prematurity. N Engl J Med. 2011;364(7):603–15.

24. Travassos A, Teixeira S, Ferreira P, et al. Intravitreal bevacizumab in aggressive posterior retinopathy of prematurity. Ophthalmic Surg Lasers Imaging. 2007;38:233–7.

25. Quiroz-Mercado H, Martinez-Castellanos MA, Hernandez-Rojas ML, Salazar-Teran N, Chan RV. Antiangiogenic therapy with intravitreal bevacizumab for retinopathy of prematurity. Retina. 2008;28(Suppl):S19–25.

26. Lalwani GA, Berrocal AM, Murray TG, et al. Off-label use of intravitreal bevacizumab (Avastin) for salvage treatment in progressive threshold retinopathy of prematurity. Retina. 2008;28(Suppl): S13–8. Retina. 2009;29:127. Erratum.

27. Kusaka S, Shima C, Wada K, et al. Efficacy of intravitreal injection of bevacizumab for severe retinopathy of prematurity: a pilot study. Br J Ophthalmol. 2008;92:1450–5.

28. Dorta P, Kychenthal A. Treatment of type 1 retinopathy of prematurity with intravitreal bevacizumab (Avastin). Retina. 2010;30(Suppl):S24–31.

29. Greven CM, Tasman WS. Scleral buckling in stages 4B and 5 retinopathy of prematurity. Ophthalmol: J AAO, 97(6);817–20.

30. Trese MT. Ophthalmology. 1994;101(1):23–6. Scleral buckling for retinopathy of prematurity.

31. Hinz BJ, de Juan E Jr. Repka MX Scleral buckling surgery for active stage 4A retinopathy of prematurity. Ophthalmology. 1998;105(10):1827–30.

32. Chuang YC, Yang CM. Scleral buckling for stage 4 retinopathy of prematurity. Ophthalmic Surg Lasers. 2000;31(5):374–9.

33. Hartnett ME, Maguluri S, Thompson HW, McColm JR. Comparison of retinal outcomes after scleral buckle or lens-sparing vitrectomy for stage 4 retinopathy of prematurity. Retina. 2004;24(5):753–7.

34. Sears JE, Sonnie C. Anatomic success of lens-sparing vitrectomy with and without scleral buckle for stage 4 retinopathy of prematurity. Am J Ophthalmol. 2007;143(5):810–3.

35. Trese MT, Retinopathy of prematurity. pp 189-193. Shapiro MJ, Biglan AW, Miller MT. In: Proceedings of the international conference on retinopathy of prematurity. Chicago, IL, USA: Kugler Publications; 1993. ISBN 90 6299 1254.

36. Chow DR, Ferrone PJ, Trese MT. Refractive changes associated with scleral buckling and division in retinopathy of prematurity. Arch Ophthalmol. 1998;116(11):1446–8.

37. Wiegand W, Kroll P. Retinopathy of prematurity. pp 197–199. Shapiro MJ, Biglan AW, Miller MT. In: Proceedings of the international conference on retinopathy of prematurity. Chicago, IL, USA: Kugler Publications; 1993. ISBN 90 6299 1254.

38. Gadkari S, Kamdar R, Kulkarni S, Deshpande M, Taras S. Vision development over an extended follow-up period in babies after successful vitrectomy for stage 4b retinopathy of prematurity. Graefes Arch Clin Exp Ophthalmol.

39. Singh R, Kumari N, Katoch D, Sanghi G, Gupta A, Dogra MR. Outcome of 23-gauge pars plana vitrectomy for pediatric vitreoretinal conditions. J Pediatr Ophthalmol Strabismus. 2014;51(1):27–31.

40. Wu WC, Lai CC, Lin RI, Wang NK, Chao AN, Chen KJ, Chen TL, Hwang YS. Modified 23-gauge vitrectomy system for stage 4 retinopathy of prematurity. Arch Ophthalmol. 2011;129(10):1326–31.

41. Iwahashi-Shima C, Miki A, Hamasaki T, Otori Y, Matsushita K, Kiuchi Y, Okada M, Kusaka S. Intraocular pressure elevation is a delayed-onset complication after successful vitrectomy for stages 4 and 5 retinopathy of prematurity. Retina. 2012;32(8):1636–42.

42. Xu Y, Zhang Q, Kang X, Zhu Y, Li J, Chen Y, Zhao P. Early vitreoretinal surgery on vascularly active stage 4 retinopathy of prematurity through the preoperative intravitreal bevacizumab injection. Acta Ophthalmol. 2013;91(4):e304–10.

43. Lakhanpal RR, Fortun JA, Chan-Kai B, Holz ER. Lensectomy and vitrectomy with and without intravitreal triamcinolone acetonide for vascularly active stage 5 retinal detachments in retinopathy of prematurity. Retina. 2006;26(7):736–40.

44. Shah PK, Narendran V, Kalpana N. Triamcinolone acetonide-assisted vitrectomy for stage 4 retinopathy of prematurity. Int Ophthalmol. 2011;31(3):237–8.

45. Margherio AR, Margherio RR, Hartzer M, et al. Plasmin enzyme-assisted vitrectomy in traumatic pediatric macular holes. Ophthalmology. 1998;105:1617–20.

46. Tsukahara Y, Honda S, Imai H, et al. Autologous plasminassisted vitrectomy for stage 5 retinopathy of prematurity: a preliminary trial. Am J Ophthalmol. 2007;144:139–41.

47. Wu WC, Drenser KA, Lai M, et al. Plasmin enzyme-assisted vitrectomy for primary and reoperated eyes with stage 5 retinopathy of prematurity. Retina. 2008;28:S75–80.

48. Wong SC, Capone A Jr. Microplasmin (ocriplasmin) in pediatric vitreoretinal surgery: update and review. Retina. 2013;33(2):339–48.

49. Honda S, Hirabayashi H, Tsukahara Y, Negi A. Acute contraction of the proliferative membrane after intravitreal injection of bevacizumab for advanced retinopathy of prematurity. Graefes Arch Clin Exp Ophthalmol. 2008;246:1061–3.

Stage 5 Retinopathy of Prematurity

10

Eric Nudleman and Antonio Capone Jr

Keywords

Retinopathy of prematurity (ROP) · Childhood blindness · Leukocoria · Tractional retinal detachments · Ocriplasmin · Stage 5 detachment

Introduction

Stage 5 represents the most advanced stage of retinopathy of prematurity (ROP). Children present with a total retinal detachment, limited or no vision, and oftentimes with leukocoria due to the visibility of fibrous proliferation immediately posterior to the lens. As a result, the disease was first described with the term "retrolental fibroplasia" [1]. Since that time, we have learned a great deal about this blinding condition. Here we will review the pathogenesis, management, and prevention of stage 5 ROP.

Epidemiology of Advanced ROP

Blindness from ROP varies from country to country, primarily dependent on the level of development that allows for survival of premature babies. The World Health Organization estimates that over 50,000 children worldwide are blind from ROP [2]. The highest proportion of childhood blindness from ROP is currently in developing countries (as ranked by the United Nation Development Programme on the basis of their Human Development Index) [3]. In highly industrialized nations, where the infant mortality rate is low (<9/1000 live births), the rate of blindness from ROP is 10% [2]. In countries with high infant mortality rates (above 60/1000), the rate of ROP-related blindness is extremely low, since children are unlikely to survive to the age when ROP develops. In "middle-income" nations, however, where infant mortality rates are between 9/1000 and 60/1000, ROP is a major cause of childhood blindness, with rates approaching 40% [3].

This alarming trend has been referred to as the "third epidemic" of ROP [3]. The "first epidemic" occurred in the 1940s and 1950s in the United States, and is partially attributable to unregulated supplemental oxygen. The "second epidemic" began in the 1970s in industrialized nations, as a result of higher survival rates of extremely premature infants. Landmark clinical trials, including the Multicenter Trail of Cryotherapy for Retinopathy of Prematurity (conducted 1986–1988) [4] and the Early Treatment for Retinopathy of Prematurity Randomized Trial (conducted 1999–2002) [5], have since

E. Nudleman
Department of Ophthalmology, Shiley Eye Institute, University of California, 9415 Campus Point Drive, #0946, La Jolla, San Diego, CA 92093, USA
e-mail: eric.nudleman@gmail.com

A. Capone Jr (✉)
Department of Opthalmology, Associated Retinal Consultants, William Beaumont School of Medicine, Oakland University, 3535 W 13 Mile Rd. Suite 344, Royal Oak, MI 48073, USA
e-mail: acaponejr@yahoo.com

© Springer International Publishing AG 2017
Andrés Kychenthal B. and Paola Dorta S. (eds.), *Retinopathy of Prematurity*,
DOI 10.1007/978-3-319-52190-9_10

demonstrated that peripheral ablation in high-risk infants reduces the risk of ROP-related blindness by approximately half, paving the way for universal screening programs in most industrialized nations.

Today, the rate of stage 5 detachments in countries with universal screening is low. In the United States, the incidence of any stage of ROP is estimated to be between 1 in 511 and 1 in 820 live births [6, 7]. Among them, roughly 10% require laser photocoagulation, and 0.5% require surgical intervention. The vast majority of children in the United States that require surgery for ROP detachments are stage 4. However, the third epidemic has given rise to a considerable increase in the incidence of stage 5 detachments worldwide, necessitating further research into effective methods of prevention and treatment.

Pathogenesis

Predominantly tractional retinal detachments in ROP occur due to formation of fibrous proliferation along the ridge tissue and extending into the overlying vitreous. The vitreous sheets act as scaffolds for the extension of the fibrotic tissue. Contraction occurs along various vectors, most commonly toward the center of the eye, as well as posterior toward the optic nerve or anterior toward the lens. The tractional vectors can be summarized as (i) intrinsic to the retina, (ii) ridge to lens, (iii) ridge to ridge, (iv) ridge to ciliary body, (v) ridge to retina, and (vi) persistent stalk tissue (Fig. 10.1). Without intervention, an eye with progressive cicatricial traction will ultimately completely detach (Fig. 10.2). The configuration of a stage 5 funnel-shaped detachment can be further described as open or closed anteriorly, and open or closed posteriorly. Late stage 5 presents typically present with leukocoria due to a dense opaque fibrovascular plaque posterior to the crystalline lens (Fig. 10.3).

A persistent hyaloidal vasculature is common in eyes of premature infants that progress to late stages of ROP, despite appropriate laser photocoagulation. Evidence from the oxygen-induced

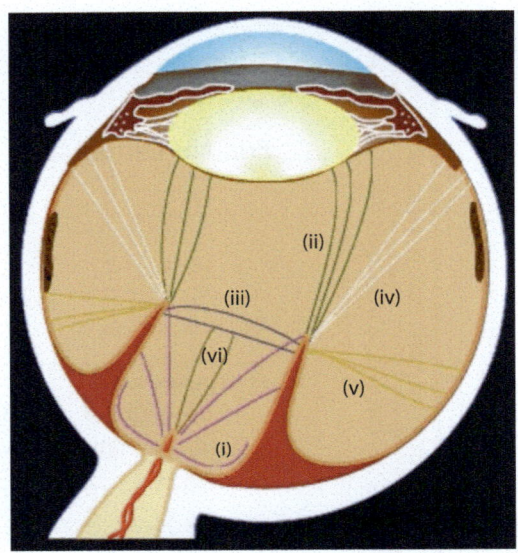

Fig. 10.1 Schematic demonstrating the tractional vectors in advanced retinopathy of prematurity, including (*i*) intrinsic to the retina, (*ii*) ridge to lens, (*iii*) ridge to ridge, (*iv*) ridge to ciliary body, (*v*) ridge to retina, and (*vi*) persistent stalk tissue

retinopathy (OIR) murine model, as well as human histological, biochemical, and clinical observations, provides insight into the pathophysiology of these cases. The development of the retinal vasculature in utero occurs under relatively hypoxic conditions, in which VEGF plays a critical role in driving developmental angiogenesis [8, 9]. The hyaloidal vasculature fills the developing vitreous with extensive connections to the developing retina. Systematic involution of these vessels occurs during development, beginning by 12-week gestation, and is completely regressed by 35–36-week gestation [10]. The main hyaloid trunk is the last element to undergo regression. Apoptosis is required for involution of the hyaloid vessels, and is influenced by low VEGF levels [11, 12] and elements of the Wnt signaling pathway [13, 14].

In the premature infant, exposure to high levels of VEGF driven by peripheral retinal ischemia results in reduced apoptosis of the hyaloid vessels [15]. Clinically, this is evident in a visible hyaloid structure, including the tunica vasculosa lentis, and rubeosis iridis. At the same

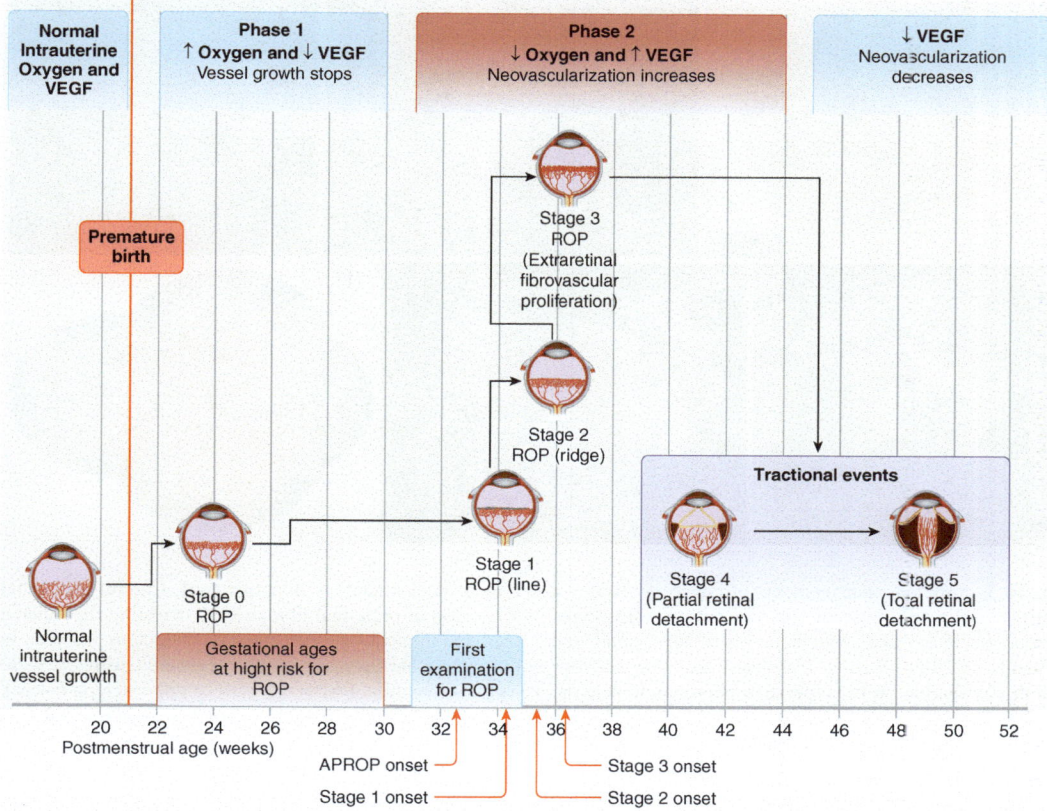

Fig. 10.2 Schematic of progression of ROP (modified from [58]). In infants born prematurely, the retina is incompletely vascularized. Furthermore, premature infants are exposed to hyperoxic conditions, relative to the intrauterine environment, in order to overcome pulmonary insufficiency and prevent cerebral ischemia. This hyperoxia results in a suppression of the signals (including VEGF) required to complete vascularization of the retina (illustrated as Phase 1). The avascular retina then predisposes the eye to abnormal compensatory neovascularization when the oxygen levels are normalized (Phase 2). The disease progresses through stages that are defined by anatomic changes occurring at the border of the vascularized retina. In stage 0, arborization begins at the terminal vessels. This is followed by the development of a demarcation line in stage 1 (illustrated in *gray*), thickening of the tissue into a ridge in stage 2 (illustrated in *red*), and fibrovascular proliferation into the vitreous in stage 3. Left untreated, the fibrovascular proliferation can contract, resulting in traction on the underlying retina. These tractional forces can overpower the retinal pigment epithelium, resulting in a partial (stage 4), or complete (stage 5), detachment of the neurosensory retina. The mean postmenstrual age for the onset of each stage is illustrated in the timeline

time, an increase in plasmin enzyme from incompetent vessels results in partial liquefaction of the vitreous [16, 17]. Concomitant activation of TGFB1 contributes to excessive scar formation, causing the purse string effect wherein the retina is drawn toward the center of the eye. Ultimately, the eye succumbs to a cicatricial phase, and unchecked will present with retrolental fibroplasia [16, 18, 19].

Clinical Course

ROP is characterized by a relatively predictable timeline of progression. Initial manifestations of the disease are usually seen at approximately 32-week postmenstrual age (PMA), and the threshold for laser ablation is reached at a mean of 37-week PMA [20, 21]. Retinal detachment

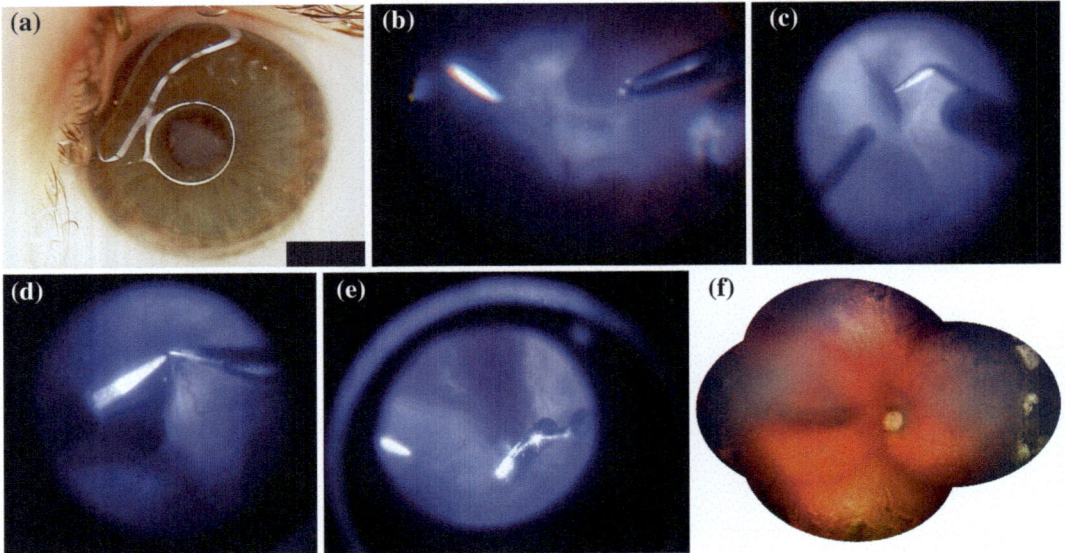

Fig. 10.3 Surgical management of stage 5 ROP. **a** RetCam color photograph of presenting phenotype. Leukocoria is evident, with a poorly dilated pupil and pigment on the anterior lens capsule. The anterior chamber is shallow. **b** Intraoperative photograph showing retrolental plaque after removal of the crystalline lens. **c** After opening the anterior plaque, the center of the funnel detachment is identified. **d** Careful bimanual dissection of preretinal fibrosis with irrigating illuminated pick and intraocular forceps. **e** The dissection proceeds to the retinal surface, and then is extended using a blunt irrigating spatula. **f** Montage RetCam photograph 6-week postoperatively demonstrating attached posterior pole

after appropriate laser ablation occurs at a mean of 41-week PMA [22]. The progression from an early stage 4A retinal detachment to stage 5 can occur quickly, often within a few weeks.

The rapidity of disease progression correlates to some degree with the level of retinal vascular activity at the time of retinal detachment. Surgery for stage 4A ROP targets interruption of transvitreal proliferative condensations. For this reason, vascular activity is rarely a reason to defer surgical intervention. In general, once surgical intervention is necessary for stage 4A ROP, earlier intervention is advisable to minimize the extent of the detachment.

In contrast, surgery for stages 4B and 5 ROP entails the mechanical removal of preretinal proliferation. An eye with a high degree of vascular activity, as represented by plus disease, florid retinal neovascularization, and rubeosis iridis, is likely to encounter significant intraoperative bleeding. In eyes with stage 4B or stage 5 detachments in the setting of significant vascularity, it is usually necessary to wait until 48–52-week PMA for vascular activity to decrease to intervene [23].

Management

The goal of ROP-related retinal detachment is to normalize anatomy in the effort to restore visual development and maximize visual potential. In stage 5 detachments, partial residual retinal detachment is common, but the goal is to remove the traction so as to reattach as much of the retina as possible and provide a stable anatomic result. To minimize the risk of creating an iatrogenic retinal tear, an anterior (translimbal) approach to lensectomy and vitrectomy is often preferable.

Various surgical approaches, including open-sky vitrectomy, two-port, and three-port vitrectomy have been utilized. Each approach has been reported with comparable success rates [24–28], leaving the preference of the surgeon dictating the technique of choice. All approaches share the goal of removing the fibrotic preretinal

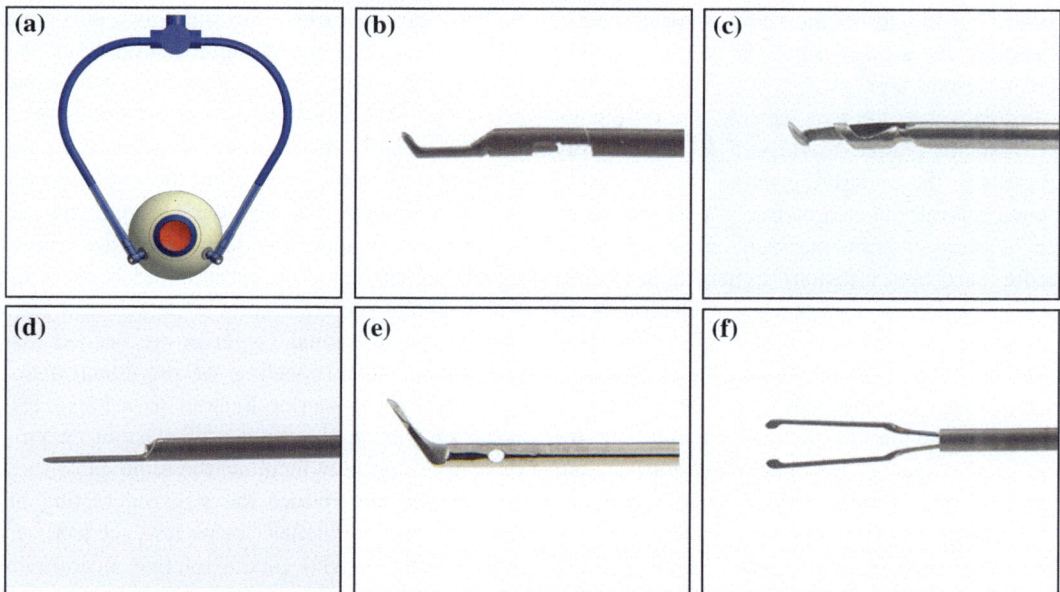

Fig. 10.4 Synergetics (O'Fallon, MO, USA) instrument design for use in pediatric vitreoretinal surgery. **a** Illustration of assembly of the combined 20/23 ga two ports infusing instrument canula system. Infusion is provided through two 20 ga canulas with embedded 23 ga instrument cannulas. The lengths of trocar blade, cannula shaft, and infusion shaft have been adjusted for smaller anatomy. **b** 23 ga Trese spatula with short platform, allowing canula compatible entry and removal. **c** 23 ga vertical forceps, with broad platform to allow dual function as dissection spatula and forceps. **d** 23 ga illuminated Capone/Rizzo Pick. Semi-malleable material allows pick to be bent to desired angle. **e** Large platform irrigating Trese Spatula. **f** Microserrated Snub Nosed Forceps. Blunt tip profile allows tissue to be engaged while preventing iatrogenic tears

material without causing iatrogenic breaks. To do so successfully, the surgery requires bimanual dissection. Instruments that aid in permitting a two-hand dissection of preretinal fibrosis have been developed. In addition to the vitrector combined with intraocular forceps, key components include an irrigating spatula, irrigating illuminated pick, and vertical forceps (Fig. 10.4).

In a two-port lensectomy–vitrectomy technique, infusion can be provided by with a 23-gauge bent butterfly needle. To avoid passing through the anteriorly drawn detached retina, entry into the eye is made immediately posterior to the limbus through the iris root, directed into the anterior lens. A two-port approach can be modified to three-port by placing an infusion canula inferotemporally immediately posterior to the limbus, to stabilize the anterior chamber and the unicameral anterior–posterior chamber

subsequently. After aspiration of the crystalline lens with the vitrector, the lens capsule is removed using intraocular forceps.

Importantly, the goals of lensectomy in such a situation differ from those of the removal of an uncomplicated congenital cataract. The benefits of preserving capsular support for potential secondary intraocular lens implantation in the future are outweighed by the likelihood of residual capsule serving as a scaffold for preretinal proliferation and circumferential vitreoretinal contraction. Once the residual capsule and the ciliary body are drawn into a contractile anterior ring, the ensuing hypotony may be difficult to treat both because the anterior contractile ring is difficult to visualize and safely dissect and because the ciliary body sustains permanent injury. Despite lenticuloretinal apposition in many stage 5 eyes, capsular material can generally be stripped away from the fibrous proliferation extending anteriorly from the retina without causing retinal breaks.

In contrast to the lens capsule, the retrolental fibrovascular plaque in stage 5 ROP is tightly adherent to the underlying retina. The plaque is opened centrally in an area free of adherent retina with a sharp instrument, such as the 23-gauge needle used for infusion, a microvitreoretinal (MVR) blade, or a 26-gauge needle on a Tb syringe can be used to initiate the dissection. Using two sharp instruments, one in each hand, a cross-action maneuver can create an opening in the plaque without causing traction on the peripheral retina. A lamellar dissection separating the plaque from the subjacent retina can then begin using an irrigating spatula and forceps, allowing a two-handed technique (see Fig. 10.3). Layers of preretinal fibrosis and vitreous are carefully removed to safely dissect down to the retinal surface. During the anterior dissection, the operating microscope is sufficient to provide illumination. As the dissection proceeds posteriorly, the illumination can be provided by either endoillumination (light pipe or illuminated pick), or by external illumination with the light pipe directed by an assistant through a hand-held irrigating contact lens.

Viscoelastic substances, such as healon, can also be used to aid in dissection. Injection of viscoelastic can be effective in separating tight retinal folds and proliferative tissue. In addition, viscoelastic is effective at stabilizes the highly mobile retinal surface, allowing dissection while preventing iatrogenic breaks. Care must be taken while injecting viscoelastic to avoid causing peripheral dialysis or posterior tears. At the conclusion of the dissection, a partial air–healon exchange is typically performed and sclerotomies are sutured.

Enzymatic Targeting of the Vitreoretinal Junction

A subset of advanced ROP surgeries fails due to incomplete removal of the posterior hyaloid. The posterior hyaloidal contraction syndrome is perhaps the most direct example, as a persistent vitreoretinal adhesion combined with hyaloidal contraction is relieved by successful vitreoretinal separation [29]. Plasmin enzyme, either the intact protein procured from blood obtained from the patient (autologous) or a parent (heterologous) or the recombinant fragment ocriplasmin (Jetrea), can be administered to cleave the vitreoretinal adhesions, mediated by laminin and fibronectin, and facilitate posterior vitreous detachment [30–32]. When additional surgeries are needed that require successful peeling of preretinal membranes or the posterior hyaloid to achieve primary surgical goals, the use of plasmin enzyme or ocriplasmin may facilitate the removal of such membranes and reduce the risk of creating an iatrogenic retinal breaks (for review, see [33]). In young children who cannot tolerate an intravitreal injection in the clinic, plasmin is injected into the vitreous cavity following induction of general anesthesia, and surgery is initiated approximately 30 min thereafter.

Outcomes

Retinal detachments in children who are properly screened and appropriately ablated are fortunately rare. However, a retinal detachment in infancy can profoundly impact visual development. Even in eyes with minor degrees of detachment, the outcomes can be poor [22, 34, 35]. As one might expect, the success rates and the visual outcomes are worse with more advanced stages of disease. Successful reattachment has been reported in 74–91% of stage 4A detachments [36–41], 62–92% of stage 4B detachments [37, 39, 41–44], and 22–48% of stage 5 detachments [24, 27, 45–47]. Visual outcomes in successful repair of stage 4A detachment can be expected to be 20/80 or better [37, 48, 49], ambulatory vision following stage 4B repair [44], and form vision following stage 5 repair [25, 50]. A summary of the outcomes of the following stage 5 repairs is shown in Table 10.1.

Surgery for stage 5 detachments is indeed challenging, with difficult and time-consuming delamination of fibrosis and zero tolerance for iatrogenic breaks. Second surgeries in advanced

Table 10.1 Summary of the outcomes of the following stage 5 repair

Study	N (Eyes)	Surgery	% Anatomic success*	VA outcomes (%)
Trese 1986 [24]	85	LV	48.2	BTL (63.4)[+++] F/F (43.9) Grasping behavior (37.5) Recognize shapes (15)
Hirose 1992 [59]	524	OSV	39.2	NA
Hirose 1993 [28]	55	OSV	100**	20/100-20/400 (7.3) 20/400-20/800 (20) 20/800-20/1600 (30.9) ≤20/3200 (41.8) LP (9.1)
Choi 1994 [60]	38	LV	29	F/F (18.4) LP (39.5) NLP (42.1)
Mintz-Hittner 1997 [25]	45	SB with subsequent LV	26.4	20/80 (11.1) 20/200 (11.1) 20/400 (22.2) 20/800 (33.3) 20/1600 (22.2)
Hartnett 2003 [54]	6	NA	50	Avg TAC score 12 (attached) Avg TAC score 6 (detached) Avg LPP score 5 (attached) Avg LPP score 2 (detached)
Cusick 2006 [27]	608	LV (94%)***	33	>20/200 (2) 5/200-20/200 (2) HM (10) LP (59) NLP (26)
Lakhanpal 2006 [61]	33	LSV	45.5	NA
Lakhanpal 2006 [46]	21	LV	28.6	NA
Wu 2008 [62]	80	Plasmin-assisted LV (83.8%)[+]	68.8	Pattern vision (7.5) F/F (3.8) LP (70) NLP (13.8) VEP positive (5)
Kondo 2009 [63]	82	LV	81.7%[++]	>20/200 (1.8) 20/200-20/2000 (11.1) FWM (14.8) LP or HM (35.2) NLP or ND (37.0)
Shah 2009 [64]	14	LV	14.3	LP (21.4) NLP (78.6)
Total	1591		38.3[#]	

OSV (open-sky vitrectomy), LV (lensectomy–vitrectomy), V (vitrectomy), LSV (lens-sparing vitrectomy), SB (scleral buckle), TAC (teller acuity cards), LPP (light perception/projection) scale, F/F (fix and follow), FWM (following with or without nystagmus), ND (not determined attributable to mental disability and/or amblyopic status), NA (not available)

*Total or partial retinal reattachment

**Study evaluated vision in eyes with successful reattachment after OSV

***100% of eyes had a vitrectomy in this study, 94% had LV. The details of the remaining 6% are not reported

[+]100% of eyes had a vitrectomy in this study, 83.8% had LV. 73/80 eyes in this study were second surgeries

[++]All eyes in this study were successfully attached. 22% of eyes had late re-detachments

[+++]Vision in this study was only tested in patients with anatomic success

[#] Hirose 1993 and Kondo 2009 excluded

cases are common. Complete retinal attachment and restoration of normal posterior pole anatomy are uncommon. Visual development following repair is typically slow and limited, with the full impact not apparent for 2 years or more. Even with good anatomic results, vision may be limited by incomplete maturation of the visual system or other neurologic comorbidities. Integration of a team to provide aggressive refractive therapy and visual rehabilitation after surgery is axiomatic. The realization that optimizing visual outcome requires much more than surgery is a great challenge to parents' wherewithal.

Why then should we continue to perform these operations? First, with the alternative being observation alone, there is a near guarantee of total blindness [1, 51]. With surgical intervention, the potential for any vision is worth proceeding. In fact, the possibility for good visual outcome with surgery exists, with letter reading vision in some cases [25, 26, 28, 52, 53]. Even in cases of very limited vision, it has been demonstrated that children can use their vision remarkably well, oftentimes ambulating with vision below the 5/200 threshold in adults [52, 54]. Finally, efforts to restore the normal anatomy provide the potential for alternative vision technologies in the future. With several devices already in clinical use (for review, see [55]), it is reasonable to assume that such devices may be applied to improving vision if anatomy permits after surgery for advanced ROP.

Screening and Prevention

It has been well demonstrated that appropriate screening of premature children, and treatment by peripheral ablative therapy, significantly reduces the risk of unfavorable anatomic and visual outcomes. The 15-year follow-up of the CRYO-ROP reported that ablative therapy reduced unfavorable structural outcomes from 48 to 27%, and reduced unfavorable visual outcomes from 62 to 44% [56]. The indications for treatment were redefined by ET-ROP, which also confirmed the efficacy of ablative therapy [5].

Available evidence suggests that improper screening, rather than improper treatment, is the cause of the majority of blindness due to ROP. Current screening guidelines in the United States specify that examinations are performed after pupillary dilation using binocular indirect ophthalmoscopy [57]. However, research is now underway to investigate the efficacy of remote digital fundus imaging (discussed in detail in a separate chapter). Advantages of RDFI include objective documentation, expert review, and potential for objective measurements of plus disease. Ultimately, efforts to improve screening promise to prevent unnecessary progression of any child, potentially worldwide, to advanced stages of ROP.

Conclusions

Stage 5 ROP represents one of the most challenging diseases in ophthalmology. Over the last few decades, dissemination of information delineating the variable clinical features of the ROP, refined screening and treatment paradigms based on evidence based studies, transition to laser from cryopexy for retinal ablation, and early lens-sparing vitreous surgery for macula-sparing partial retinal detachment (stage 4A) have mitigated the impact of advanced ROP. However, progression to retinal detachment occurs even with state-of-the-art care. Advanced ROP remains a significant problem in the United States and abroad.

The untreated natural history of stage 5 ROP is poor. Spontaneous reattachment is rare and "no light perception" blindness is all too common. Yet with experienced surgical intervention, poor visual outcomes are not invariable. It is clear that every effort must be made employing established paradigms—diligent screening, timely laser, prompt intervention for stage 4A ROP—to interrupt the pathogenetic process of ROP before eyes reach a point of no return, and normal vision is unattainable. Nevertheless, unwelcome though it is, stage 5 ROP is here to stay. Surgeons and parents have no choice but to consider the variables pertinent to undertaking surgery in a given infant, in much of the same fashion as is done with surgery for severe ocular trauma, bleb-related endophthalmitis and other poor prognosis conditions. Who can presume to know what vision restorative technologies will be available during the lifetime of an infant born today? It is reasonable to expect more options will await a sighted child than one who does not perceive light.

References

1. Terry TL. Extreme prematurity and fibroblastic overgrowth of persistent vascular sheath behind each crystalline lens. Am J Ophthalmol. 1942.
2. Gilbert C. Retinopathy of prematurity: a global perspective of the epidemics, population of babies at risk and implications for control. 2008;84:77–82. doi:10.1016/j.earlhumdev.2007.11.009.
3. Gilbert C, Rahi J, Eckstein M, et al. Retinopathy of prematurity in middle-income countries. Lancet. 1997;350:12–4. doi:10.1016/S0140-6736(97)01107-0.
4. Cryotherapy for Retinopathy of Prematurity Cooperative Group. Multicenter trial of cryotherapy for retinopathy of prematurity. Preliminary results. Arch Ophthalmol. 1988;106:471–79.
5. Early Treatment for Retinopathy of Prematurity Cooperative Group. Revised indications for the treatment of retinopathy of prematurity: results of the early treatment for retinopathy of prematurity randomized trial. Arch Ophthalmol. 2003;121:1684–94. doi:10.1001/archopht.121.12.1684.
6. Chiang MF, Arons RR, Flynn JT, Starren JB. Incidence of retinopathy of prematurity from 1996 to 2000: analysis of a comprehensive New York state patient database. Ophthalmology. 2004;111:1317–25. doi:10.1016/j.ophtha.2003.10.030.
7. Lad EM, Nguyen TC, Morton JM, Moshfeghi DM. Retinopathy of prematurity in the United States. Br J Ophthalmol. 2008;92:320–5. doi:10.1136/bjo.2007.126201.
8. Chan-Ling T, Gock B, Stone J. The effect of oxygen on vasoformative cell division. Evidence that "physiological hypoxia" is the stimulus for normal retinal vasculogenesis. Invest Ophthalmol Vis Sci. 1995;36:1201–14.
9. Stone J, Itin A, Alon T, et al. Development of retinal vasculature is mediated by hypoxia-induced vascular endothelial growth factor (VEGF) expression by neuroglia. J Neurosci. 1995;15:4738–47.
10. Zhu M, Madigan MC, van Driel D, et al. The human hyaloid system: cell death and vascular regression.
11. Exp Eye Res. 2000;70:767–76. doi:10.1006/exer.2000.0844.
11. Stahl A, Connor KM, Sapieha P, et al. The mouse retina as an angiogenesis model. Invest Ophthalmol Vis Sci. 2010;51:2813–26. doi:10.1167/iovs.10-5176.
12. Penn JS, Tolman BL, Lowery LA. Variable oxygen exposure causes preretinal neovascularization in the newborn rat. Invest Ophthalmol Vis Sci. 1993;34:576–85.
13. Lobov IB, Rao S, Carroll TJ, et al. WNT7b mediates macrophage-induced programmed cell death in patterning of the vasculature. Nature. 2005;437:417–21. doi:10.1038/nature03928.
14. Liu C, Nathans J. An essential role for frizzled 5 in mammalian ocular development. Development. 2008;135:3567–76. doi:10.1242/dev.028076.
15. Alon T, Hemo I, Itin A, et al. Vascular endothelial growth factor acts as a survival factor for newly formed retinal vessels and has implications for retinopathy of prematurity. Nat Med. 1995;1:1024–8.
16. Flaumenhaft R, Abe M, Mignatti P, Rifkin DB. Basic fibroblast growth factor-induced activation of latent transforming growth factor beta in endothelial cells: regulation of plasminogen activator activity. J Cell Biol. 1992;118:901–9.
17. Hikichi T, Nomiyama G, Nomiyama G, et al. Vitreous changes after treatment of retinopathy of prematurity. 1999;43:543–5.
18. Sato Y, Rifkin DB. Inhibition of endothelial cell movement by pericytes and smooth muscle cells: activation of a latent transforming growth factor-beta 1-like molecule by plasmin during co-culture. J Cell Biol. 1989;109:309–15.
19. Mandriota SJ, Menoud PA, Pepper MS. Transforming growth factor beta 1 down-regulates vascular endothelial growth factor receptor 2/flk-1 expression in vascular endothelial cells. J Biol Chem. 1996;271:11500.
20. Palmer EA, Flynn JT, Hardy RJ, et al. Incidence and early course of retinopathy of prematurity. The Cryotherapy for Retinopathy of Prematurity Cooperative Group. Ophthalmology. 1991;98:1628–40.
21. Schaffer DB, Palmer EA, Plotsky DF, et al. Prognostic factors in the natural course of retinopathy of prematurity. The Cryotherapy for Retinopathy of Prematurity Cooperative Group. Ophthalmology. 1993;100:230.
22. Repka MX, Tung B, Good WV, et al. Outcome of eyes developing retinal detachment during the Early Treatment for Retinopathy of Prematurity Study (ETROP). Arch Ophthalmol. 2006;124:24–30. doi:10.1001/archopht.124.1.24.
23. Hartnett ME. Features associated with surgical outcome in patients with stages 4 and 5 retinopathy of prematurity. Retina (Philadelphia, Pa). 2003;23:322–29.
24. Trese MT. Visual results and prognostic factors for vision following surgery for stage V retinopathy of prematurity. Ophthalmology. 1986;93:574–9.

25. Mintz-Hittner HA, O'Malley RE, Kretzer FL. Long-term form identification vision after early, closed, lensectomy-vitrectomy for stage 5 retinopathy of prematurity. Ophthalmology. 1997;104:454–9.

26. Fuchino Y, Hayashi H, Kono T, Ohshima K. Long-term follow up of visual acuity in eyes with stage 5 retinopathy of prematurity after closed vitrectomy. Am J Ophthalmol. 1995;120:308–16.

27. Cusick M, Charles MK, AGR NE, et al. Anatomical and visual results of vitreoretinal surgery for stage 5 retinopathy of prematurity. Retina. 2006;26:729–35. doi:10.1097/01.iae.0000244268.21514.f7.

28. Hirose T, Katsumi O, Mehta MC, Schepens CL. Vision in stage 5 retinopathy of prematurity after retinal reattachment by open-sky vitrectomy. Arch Ophthalmol. 1993;111:345–9.

29. Joshi MM, Trese MT, CAPONE A Jr. Optical coherence tomography findings in stage 4A retinopathy of prematurity. Ophthalmology. 2006;113:657–60. doi:10.1016/j.ophtha.2006.01.007.

30. Kohno T, Sorgente N, Ishibashi T, et al. Immunofluorescent studies of fibronectin and laminin in the human eye. Invest Ophthalmol Vis Sci. 1987;28:506–14.

31. Gandorfer A. Objective of pharmacologic vitreolysis. Dev Ophthalmol. 2009;44:1. doi:10.1159/000223938.

32. Liotta LA, Goldfarb RH, Brundage R, et al. Effect of plasminogen activator (urokinase), plasmin, and thrombin on glycoprotein and collagenous components of basement membrane. Cancer Res. 1981;41:4629–36.

33. Wong SC, Jr CAPONEA. Microplasmin (Ocriplasmin) in pediatric vitreoretinal surgery. Retina. 2013;33:339–48. doi:10.1097/IAE.0b013e31826e86e0.

34. Gilbert WS, Quinn GE, Dobson V, et al. Partial retinal detachment at 3 months after threshold retinopathy of prematurity. Long-term structural and functional outcome. Multicenter Trial of Cryotherapy for Retinopathy of Prematurity Cooperative Group. Arch Ophthalmol. 1996;114:1085–91.

35. Repka MX, Tung B, Good WV, et al. Outcome of eyes developing retinal detachment during the early treatment for retinopathy of prematurity study. Arch Ophthalmol. 2011;129:1175–9. doi:10.1001/archophthalmol.2011.229.

36. Capone A, Trese MT. Lens-sparing vitreous surgery for tractional stage 4A retinopathy of prematurity retinal detachments. Ophthalmology. 2001;108:2068–70.

37. Hubbard GB III, Cherwick DH, Burian G. Lens-sparing vitrectomy for stage 4 retinopathy of prematurity. Ophthalmology. 2004;111:2274–2277. e1. doi:10.1016/j.ophtha.2004.05.030.

38. Moshfeghi AA, Awner S, Salam GA, Ferrone PJ. Excellent visual outcome and reversal of dragging after lens sparing vitrectomy for progressive tractional stage 4a retinopathy of prematurity retinal detachment. Retina (Philadelphia, Pa) 2004;4:615–16.

39. Lakhanpal RR, Sun RL, Albini TA, Holz ER. Anatomic success rate after 3-port lens-sparing vitrectomy in stage 4A or 4B retinopathy of prematurity. Ophthalmology. 2005;112:1569–73. doi:10.1016/j.ophtha.2005.03.031.

40. Bhende P, Gopal L, Sharma T, et al. Functional and anatomical outcomes after primary lens-sparing pars plana vitrectomy for Stage 4 retinopathy of prematurity. Indian J Ophthalmol. 2009;57:267. doi:10.4103/0301-4738.53050.

41. Singh R, Reddy DM, Barkmeier AJ, et al. Long-term visual outcomes following lens-sparing vitrectomy for retinopathy of prematurity. Br J Ophthalmol. 2012;96:1395–8. doi:10.1136/bjophthalmol-2011-301353.

42. Yu YS, Kim S-J, Kim SY, et al. Lens-sparing vitrectomy for stage 4 and stage 5 retinopathy of prematurity. Korean J Ophthalmol. 2006;20:113–7.

43. Choi J, Kim JH, Kim S-J, Yu YS. Long-term results of lens-sparing vitrectomy for stages 4B and 5 retinopathy of prematurity. Korean J Ophthalmol. 2011;25:305–10. doi:10.3341/kjo.2011.25.5.305.

44. Rayes El EN, Vinekar A, Capone A. Three-year anatomic and visual outcomes after vitrectomy for stage 4B retinopathy of prematurity. Retina (Philadelphia, Pa) 2008;28:568–572. doi:10.1097/IAE.0b013e3181610f97.

45. Gopal L, Sharma T, Shanmugam M, et al. Surgery for stage 5 retinopathy of prematurity: the learning curve and evolving technique. Indian J Ophthalmol. 2000;48:101–6.

46. Lakhanpal RR, Fortun JA, Chan-Kai B, Holz ER. Lensectomy and vitrectomy with and without intravitreal triamcinolone acetonide for vascularly active stage 5 retinal detachments in retinopathy of prematurity. Retina. 2006;26:736–40. doi:10.1097/01.iae.0000244257.60524.89.

47. Trese MT. Surgical results of stage V retrolental fibroplasia and timing of surgical repair. Ophthalmology. 1984;91:461–6.

48. Prenner JL, CAPONE A Jr., Trese MT. Visual outcomes after lens-sparing vitrectomy for stage 4A retinopathy of prematurity. Ophthalmology. 2004;111:2271–73. doi:10.1016/j.ophtha.2004.06.021.

49. Lakhanpal RR. Visual outcomes after 3-Port lens-sparing vitrectomy in stage 4 retinopathy of prematurity. Arch Ophthalmol. 2006;124:675–9. doi:10.1001/archopht.124.5.675.

50. Trese MT, Droste PJ. Long-term postoperative results of a consecutive series of stages 4 and 5 retinopathy of prematurity. Ophthalmology. 1998;105:992–7. doi:10.1016/S0161-6420(98)96024-9.

51. King MJ. Retrolental fibroplasia; a clinical study of 238 cases. Arch Ophthalmol. 1950;43:694–711.

52. Seaber JH, Machemer R, Eliott D, et al. Long-term visual results of children after initially successful vitrectomy for stage V retinopathy of prematurity. Ophthalmology. 1995;102:199.

53. Kono T, Oshima K, Fuchino Y. Surgical results and visual outcomes of vitreous surgery for advanced

stages of retinopathy of prematurity. Jpn J Ophthalmol. 2000;44:661–7.

54. Hartnett ME, Rodier DW, McColm JR, Thompson HW. Long-term vision results measured with teller acuity cards and a new light perception/projection scale after management of late stages of retinopathy of prematurity. Arch Ophthalmol. 2003;121:991–6. doi:10.1001/archopht.121.7.991.

55. Chuang AT, Margo CE, Greenberg PB. Retinal implants: a systematic review. Br J Ophthalmol. 2014;. doi:10.1136/bjophthalmol-2013-303708.

56. Cryotherapy for Retinopathy of Prematurity Cooperative Group. 15-Year Outcomes Following Threshold Retinopathy of Prematurity. Arch Ophthalmol. 2005;123:311–8. doi:10.1001/archopht.123.3.311.

57. Fierson WM, American Academy of Pediatrics Section on Ophthalmology, American Academy of Ophthalmology, et al. Screening examination of premature infants for retinopathy of prematurity. Pediatrics. 2013;131:189–195. doi:10.1542/peds.2012-2996.

58. Mintz-Hittner HA, Kennedy KA, Chuang AZ, BEAT-ROP Cooperative Group. Efficacy of intravitreal bevacizumab for stage 3 + retinopathy of prematurity. N Engl J Med. 2011;364:603–15. doi:10.1056/NEJMoa1007374.

59. Hirose T, Schepens CL, Katsumi O, Mehta MC. Open-Sky vitrectomy for severe retinal detachment caused by advanced retinopathy of prematurity. Retinopathy of prematurity. New York, NY: Springer New York; 1992. p. 95–114.

60. Choi WC, Yu YS. Surgical management for stage 5 retinopathy of prematurity. Korean J Ophthalmol. 1994;8:37–41.

61. Lakhanpal RR, Sun RL, Albini TA, Holz ER. Anatomical success rate after primary three-port lens-sparing vitrectomy in stage 5 retinopathy of prematurity. Retina. 2006;26:724–8. doi:10.1097/01.iae.0000244274.95963.1e.

62. Wu W-C, Drenser KA, Lai M, et al. Plasmin enzyme-assisted vitrectomy for primary and reoperated eyes with stage 5 retinopathy of prematurity. Retina (Philadelphia, Pa). 2008;28:S75–80. doi:10.1097/IAE.0b013e318158ea0e.

63. Kondo H, Arita N, Osato M, et al. Late recurrence of retinal detachment following successful vitreous surgery for stages 4B and 5 retinopathy of prematurity. 2009;147(661–6):e1. doi:10.1016/j.ajo.2008.10.006.

64. Shah PK, Narendran V, Kalpana N, Tawansy KA. Anatomical and visual outcome of stages 4 and 5 retinopathy of prematurity. Eye. 2007;23:176–80. doi:10.1038/sj.eye.6702939.

Complications of Retinopathy of Prematurity Treatment

Wei-Chi Wu and Jane Z. Kuo

Abstract

Although major progress has been made in the management of retinopathy of prematurity (ROP), complications arising from various treatment applications are common and require careful monitoring and surveillance. In this chapter, we summarize the complications associated with the use of cryotherapy, laser photocoagulation, anti-vascular endothelial growth factor agents, scleral buckle, and vitrectomy in the treatment of ROP. While some complications are acute, others may not develop until many years later. The timing when these complications arise, during active or chronic stage, also varies. Proper management should be delivered once these complications are identified.

Keywords

Cryotherapy · Intravitreal injection · Laser photocoagulation · Retinopathy of prematurity · Scleral buckle · Vascular endothelial growth factor · Vitrectomy

Over the past several decades, significant advances in the management of retinopathy of prematurity (ROP) have led to an improved visual outcome in this once devastating blinding disorder; however, treatment-induced complications are not uncommon. Current treatments for ROP may include cryotherapy, laser photocoagulation, anti-vascular endothelial growth factor (VEGF) agents, scleral buckling, and/or vitrectomy. In general, cryotherapy, laser photocoagulation, and anti-VEGF treatments are particularly useful for Type-1 pre-threshold ROP as defined by the Early Treatment for Retinopathy of Prematurity Study (ETROP) [1] or threshold ROP. For advanced ROP (stage 4 and 5), surgical managements with scleral buckling

W.-C. Wu (✉)
Ophthalmology, Chang Gung Memorial Hospital,
No. 5, Fu-Hsin St., Kweishan, Taoyuan 333, Taiwan
e-mail: weichi666@gmail.com

J.Z. Kuo
Department of Ophthalmology, Shiley Eye Institute,
University of California, San Diego, 9415 Campus
Point Drive, La Jolla, CA 92093, USA
e-mail: janekuo@gmail.com

© Springer International Publishing AG 2017
Andrés Kychenthal B. and Paola Dorta S. (eds.), *Retinopathy of Prematurity*,
DOI 10.1007/978-3-319-52190-9_11

and/or vitrectomy are usually necessary for eyes that have progressed to retinal detachment. Understanding the complications associated with each type of treatment are of vital importance, so that postoperative monitoring may be properly performed. While some complications are transient and may require short-term monitoring, other complications may be more chronic and require longer periods of surveillance. Proper treatments should be given once these complications are identified.

Our prior study showed that patients with a history of threshold ROP are more likely to show abnormal foveal development and have poorer visual prognosis compared to other patient groups despite a fundus with no macular dragging, disc dragging, or retinal detachment [2]. A steeper corneal curvature, shallower anterior chamber, and greater lens thickness are the primary changes in the optical components in these patients [2]. It is likely that these structural changes accounted for the increased incidence of refractive errors, glaucoma, and cataract in ROP children compared to children without a history of ROP or treatment.

While some complications may occur during the active stages of ROP, others may develop sometime after the resolution of ROP. Early complications are usually associated with the reactivation of disease activities or side effects from the treatments. For examples, vitreous hemorrhage could result from the proliferation and reactivation of neovascularization or from the contraction of the fibrovascular membranes. Cataracts may result from absorption of laser energy in the lens. Retinal holes may form due to excessive laser energy used during ROP treatments. Late complications are often associated with the late effects of treatments or changes associated with eye development. For example, retinal break or retinal detachment may arise from areas previously treated with laser or cryotherapy. The retina becomes thinner after previous peripheral ablative procedures. With chronic traction from the retinal scarring due to these procedures, retinal holes typically result in retinal detachment later in the years. Retinal detachment may also develop if a retinal break is present and the vitreous becomes liquefied after prior treatments.

ROP is a lifelong disease and ROP patients with a history of treatment should be closely monitored for life [3]. Some complications may arise many years after the resolution of ROP [4]. In addition to regular follow-up, educating patients to seek professional help when visual changes occur is another area of importance.

Cryotherapy

The first demonstrated successful treatment of ROP was cryotherapy. The Multicenter Trial of Cryotherapy for ROP (CRYO-ROP) Study indicated that destruction of the peripheral retina with cryotherapy slowed progression in threshold ROP; however, this type of treatment was shown to be associated with many complications. Complications associated with unfavorable cosmetic outcomes [5] may include strabismus (12.8%), nystagmus (3.3%), total retrolental membrane (1%), epiphora (0.6%), corneal opacity (0.6%), cataract (0.3%), and episcleral hyperemia (0.3%). A comparable subgroup analysis examined at 24 months post-term showed complications of strabismus (14.4%), nystagmus (2.2%), epiphora (0.5%), corneal opacity (0.7%), cataract (0.5%), episcleral hyperemia (0.5%), lid fissure asymmetry (2.4%), and corneal diameter asymmetry (2.0%). The rate of adverse aesthetic outcome was highest in eyes that had developed more severe acute ROP and an unfavorable structural outcome.

Although results of the CRYO-ROP study showed that cryotherapy treatment was superior to natural history in the management of ROP, a number of treated eyes continued to progress to macular distortion and rhegmatogenous retinal detachment with extremely poor visual outcome (Figs. 11.1 and 11.2) [6–8]. There is a higher percentage of poor structural and functional outcomes in eyes treated with cryotherapy compared with eyes undergoing laser treatment [9]. Higher rates of systemic complications and myopia were also identified after treatment [9]. Increased postoperative inflammation was also

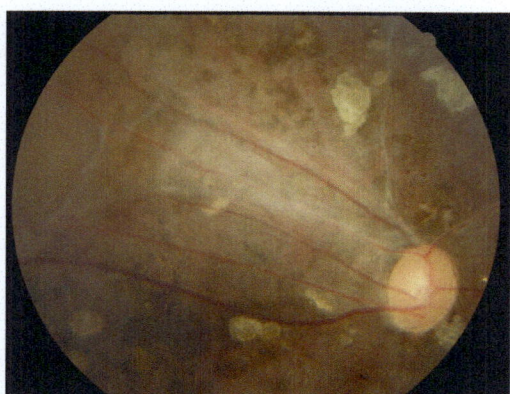

Fig. 11.1 Development of rhegmatogenous retinal detachment after treatment with cryotherapy in a case of threshold ROP. Disc dragging, diffuse retinal pigmentation, and thinning of the retina due to chronic traction are seen in the fundus. ROP = retinopathy of prematurity

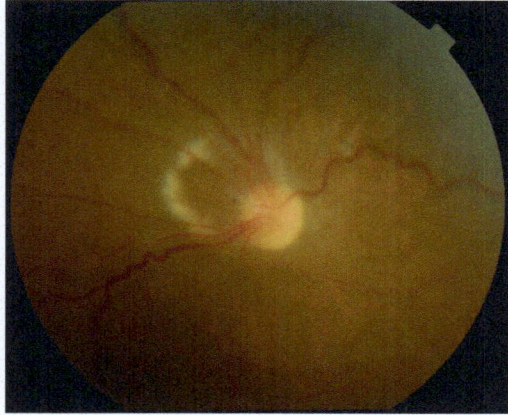

Fig. 11.2 Development of a shallow rhegmatogenous retinal detachment after treatment with cryotherapy in a case of threshold ROP. Very torturous retinal vessels as well as the subretinal exudation around the disc were noted. ROP = retinopathy of prematurity

Table 11.1 Complications associated with cryotherapy

Refractive errors
Nystagmus
Strabismus
Conjunctival scarring
Conjunctival tissue proliferation
Subconjunctival hemorrhage or edema
Conjunctival tear
Corneal opacity
Cataract
Retrolental membrane
Vitreous hemorrhage
Progression of tractional retinal detachment due to constriction of proliferative tissues
Retinal holes
Rhegmatogenous retinal detachment (Figs. 11.1 and 11.2)
Macular hole
Macular distortion

Laser Photocoagulation

Due to a higher complication rate, increased postoperative inflammation, and an unfavorable structural and functional outcome in patients treated with cryotherapy, the diode laser photocoagulation is currently regarded as the standard of treatment for the management of ROP. Despite the superior results from this procedure, complications may also arise from the use of laser treatment in the management of ROP. These complications include the absorption of laser energy in the anterior segment, lens, and the retina. Deciding on the amount of energy to use is challenging since direct laser-causing damage such as retinal breaks or retinal detachment could arise if excessive energy is used, but insufficient laser treatment could also result in skip areas and lead to reactivation of ROP (Figs. 11.3, 11.4 and 11.5) [10]. In addition, laser-induced complications also cause the peripheral retinal damage and cause strabismus, visual field constriction, and refractive errors.

noted and anti-inflammatory agents are often required post treatment. Even eyes with a favorable anatomical result had poor functional outcomes. For these reasons, this procedure is less commonly performed today. Possible complications associated with cryotherpay are shown in Table 11.1.

Table 11.2 Complications associated with laser photocoagulation

Refractive errors
Visual field constriction
Strabismus
Corneal opacity
Iris atrophy and iris synechia (due to inflammation associated with laser treatment or inadvertent damage by laser photocoagulation)
Glaucoma
Cataract
Hyphema
Vitreous hemorrhage
Progression of tractional retinal detachment (Fig. 11.4)
Retinal holes or tears (due to excessive laser energy or traction from adjacent proliferative tissue)
Rhegmatogenous retinal detachment (Fig. 11.5)
Exudative retinal detachment
Retinal vessel occlusion
Anterior ischemic syndrome
Hypotony
Phthisis

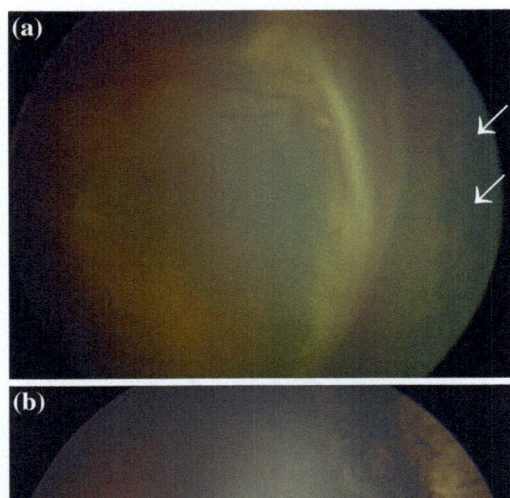

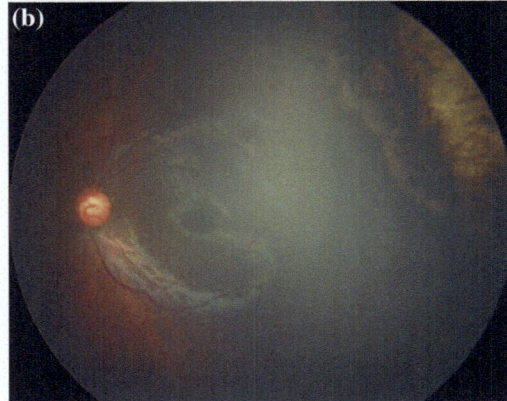

Possible complications associated with laser photocoagulation are shown in Table 11.2.

Fig. 11.3 Reactivation of ROP after laser treatment. Severe reactivation of ROP, leading to retinal detachment (**a**). Some preretinal hemorrhage was noted around the neovascular tissues. Some skip areas were noted at the peripheral retina (*white arrows*). Regressed ROP was noted in the left eye following additional laser treatment (**b**). ROP = retinopathy of prematurity

Anti-Vascular Endothelial Growth Factor Agents

Because VEGF concentrations are highly elevated in advanced ROP, a growing body of evidence supports the rationale of pharmacologic targeting of VEGF in the treatment of ROP [11–13]. Bevacizumab (Avastin; Genentech Inc., South San Francisco, CA) and ranibizumab (Lucentis; Genentech Inc., South San Francisco, CA) are two monoclonal anti-VEGF agents, with different molecular sizes, structures, and half-lives [14, 15], that have demonstrated efficacy in the treatment of type-1 ROP [16–21].

Treatment techniques with intravitreal anti-VEGF agents, such as dose, injection site, depth, and angle are modified for the pediatric population. The injection is performed with a 30-gauge needle that is initially directed along an angle that is perpendicular to the globe and then redirected slightly toward the center of the eyeball after the needle had passed the equator of the lens. These modifications mitigate or avoid damaging either the lens or the retina [21]. The injected dosages (0.625 mg/0.025 ml for bevacizumab and 0.25 mg/0.025 ml for ranibizumab) are half dose of those used in the adults. To avoid unintended complications, physicians should be familiar with the various injection techniques before applying this treatment to the newborns [21, 22]. Post injection, infants are closely monitored for potential complications, including cataract, endophthalmitis, and retinal detachment.

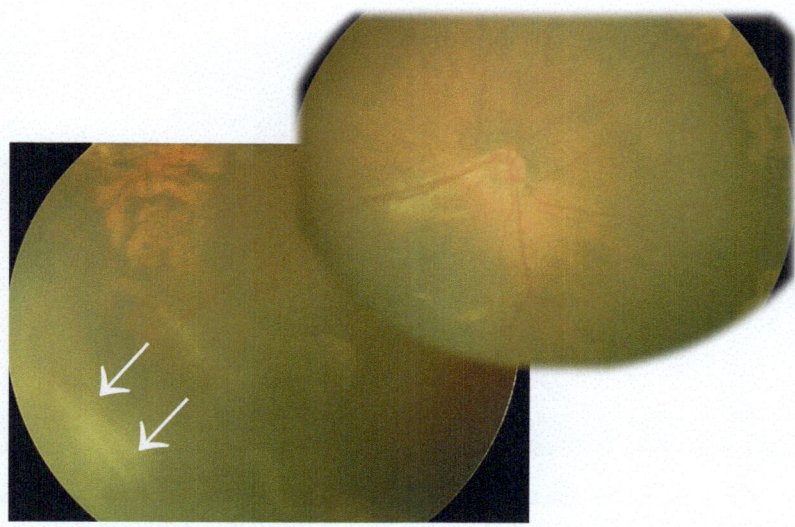

Fig. 11.4 Reactivation of ROP after laser treatment. Reactivation of ROP was noted, leading to retinal detachment (*white arrows*). ROP = retinopathy of prematurity

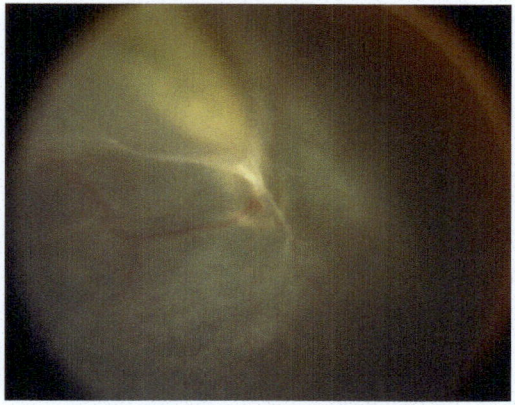

Fig. 11.5 Reactivation of ROP and progression to total retinal detachment after laser treatment. Combination of tractional and rhegmatogenous retinal detachment developed because of retinal holes on the previously lasered area. ROP = retinopathy of prematurity

Another complication with intravitreal injection of bevacizumab (IVB) in ROP is a longer recurrence time compared with conventional laser therapy. The BEAT-ROP study [18] observed a late recurrence of disease in 2 of 62 eyes in infants with zone 1 disease and in 4 of 78 eyes in infants with a posterior zone 2 disease after treatment with IVB. Considering all recurrences together, the time to recurrence was 16.0 ± 4.6 weeks in 6 eyes that received IVB injection, compared with 6.2 ± 5.7 weeks in 32 eyes that received conventional laser therapy. Additional laser photocoagulation may be necessary in these patients.

IVB may neutralize the VEGF concentration that is present in the vitreous cavity, but has no role in inhibiting continual production of VEGF in the avascular area. Thus, a late recurrence is possible if VEGF is continually produced in the avascular retina after degradation of bevacizumab and the subsequent loss of its therapeutic effects. Thus, laser therapy may still be necessary for nonresponders to IVB [21].

It has been noted that a small proportion of bevacizumab could leak into the systemic circulation following IVB injection [23, 24]. The inhibition of systemic VEGF raises concerns that these important physiological effects associated with VEGF in development [25–27] may lead to abnormal organogenesis or neurodevelopment. Sato et al. [23] found that the serum VEGF was suppressed for up to 2 weeks after IVB injection. However, Martínez-Castellanos et al. [28] did not find any abnormality in neuro-developments 5 years after the use of IVB in a longitudinal

(a)   (b)

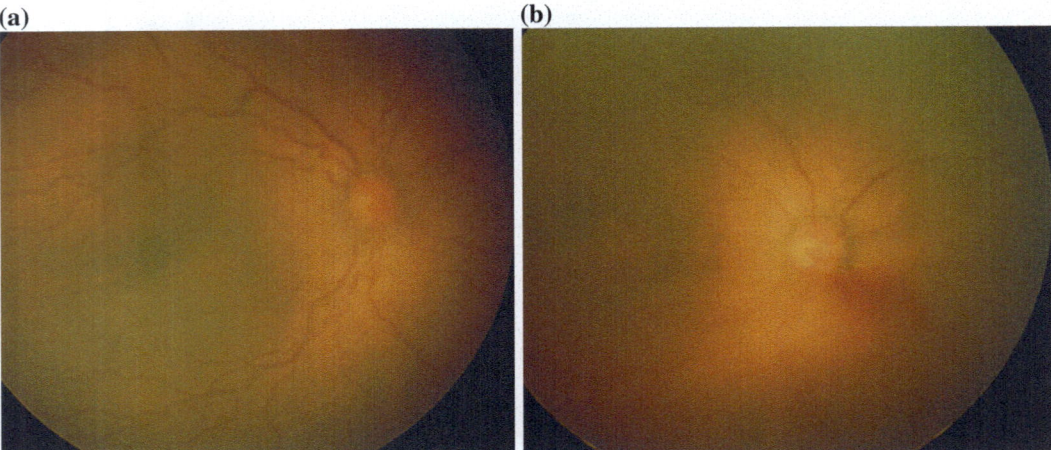

Fig. 11.6 Preretinal hemorrhage after injection of bevacizumab in the right eye of a patient with stage 3 ROP. Before injection of bevacizumab, the retinal vessels were torturous but no preretinal hemorrhage was seen (**a**).

After injection of bevacizumab, the retinal vessel tortuosity decreased but some retinal hemorrhage was present (**b**). ROP = retinopathy of prematurity

Table 11.3 Complications associated with anti-vascular endothelial growth factor agents

Progression of tractional retinal detachment due to constriction of proliferative tissues [33]
Retinal holes
Retinal detachment
Endophthalmitis
Vitreous or preretinal hemorrhage (Fig. 11.6)
Transient vascular shealthing or vessel occlusion (Fig. 11.7)
Neuro-developmental delay

refractive status with anti-VEGF agents [21, 31] compared to laser-treated patients may be due to the fact that a better preserved peripheral retina in the anti-VEGF treated eyes helps the emmetropization process. The peripheral retina has been demonstrated to be important in the regulation of emmetropization in animal models, possibly due to its visual feedback [32]. Possible complications associated with anti-vascular endothelial growth factor agents are listed in Table 11.3 and Figs. 11.6 and 11.7.

study. Banker et al. [29] also did not report signs of developmental delay 6 years following the use of IVB. However, both of these studies were limited by a modest number of patients and of a non-randomized study design. The long-term safety and systemic effects of anti-VEGF agents in the treatment of ROP remain to be clarified [30].

Another concern from treatment-induced complication is the development of myopia and worsening of refractive error in ROP patients. Harder et al. [31] reported an incidence of high myopia in 9% of patients treated with bevacizumab compared with 42% in the laser group. This relatively favorable outcomes in

Scleral Buckle

The management of retinal detachment in advanced ROP remains complicated. Scleral buckle has been proposed in the treatment of stage 4 and stage 5 ROP; however, it is generally less successful and is associated with more complications compared to the use of vitrectomy in the management of advance ROP [33, 34]. This is largely due to the fact that scleral buckle only relieves traction around the buckle area and does not relieve the tractional forces in the posterior pole. Furthermore, higher refractive errors and astigmatism are induced by the placement of a high scleral buckle in a fast growing eye. In

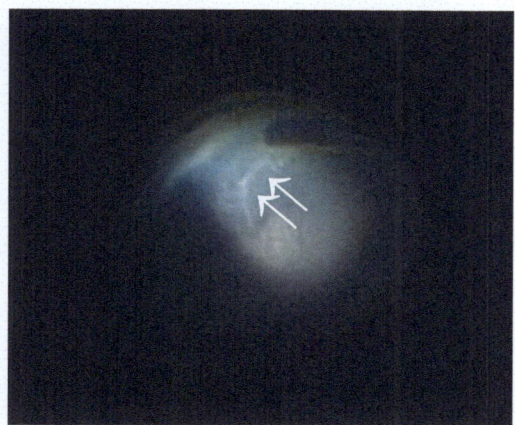

Fig. 11.7 Transient retinal vessel sheathing after injection of bevacizumab in a patient with stage 4A ROP. Three days after injection of bevacizumab, the inferior retinal vein sheathing (*arrows*) was noted during the vitrectomy surgery

Table 11.4 Complications associated with scleral buckle

Refractive errors
Astigmatism
Strabismus
Ocular muscle disruption
Conjunctival scarring
Conjunctival tissue proliferation
Sclera perforation [35]
Buckling extrusion
Deformation of the globe
Limited eye growth
Glaucoma
Cataract
Progression of tractional retinal detachment due to constriction of proliferative tissues
Retinal holes
Rhegmatogenous retinal detachment due to drainage of subretinal fluid

Table 11.5 Complications associated with vitrectomy

Refractive errors
Astigmatism
Strabismus
Conjunctival scarring
Hyphema (Fig. 11.8)
Glaucoma (Fig. 11.9)
Cataract (Figs. 11.9 and 11.10)
Preretinal or vitreous hemorrhage (Fig. 11.11)
Progression of tractional retinal detachment
Retinal holes
Rhegmatogenous retinal detachment
Endophthalmitis

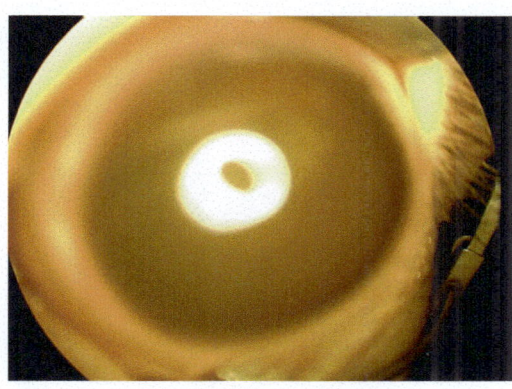

Fig. 11.8 Total hyphema after vitrectomy for ROP. Hyphema developed a few months after vitrectomy for stage 4B ROP, possibility due to bleeding and reactivation of the neovascularization in the angle. This is an indication of poor retinal condition, such as retinal re-detachment in the peripheral retina. Aggressive steroid was given to help reabsorb the blood. ROP = retinopathy of prematurity

Vitrectomy

Vitrectomy surgery for retinal detachment in advanced ROP remains challenging. Because newborn eyes are much smaller than adult eyes, the anatomy and the surgical approaches are different. Instruments should be adjusted for use in smaller eyes [35]. Most importantly, the chance to amend undesirable complications, i.e., retinal breaks, is much lower. The presence of iatrogenic breaks in stage 5 ROP during the

these incidences, it is important to section or remove the encircling buckle a few months after the initial surgery to allow for continuation of eye development in these patients. Possible complications associated with scleral buckle are listed in Table 11.4.

(a)   (b)

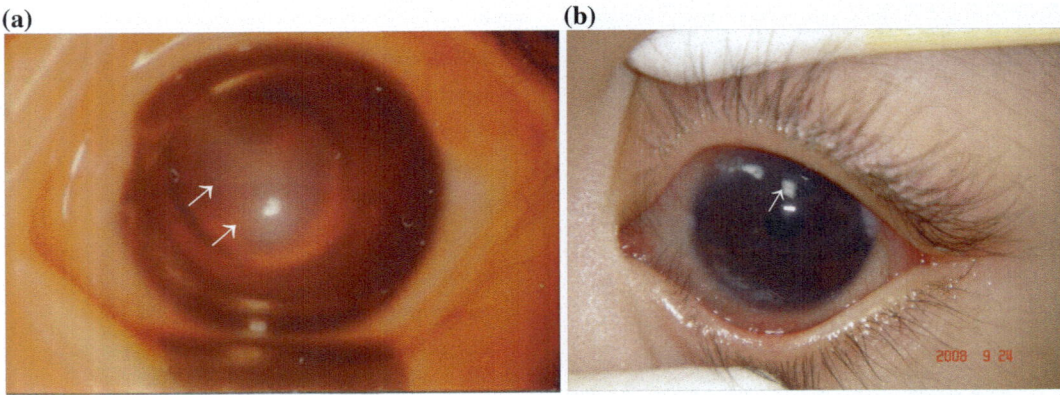

Fig. 11.9 Development of glaucoma and cataract 9 months after vitrectomy for stage 4B ROP. These complications, as well as corneal opacity (*white arrows*) were noted (**a**). After lens aspiration, trabeculectomy, and trabeculotomy, the cornea regained its clarity and the intraocular pressure was within normal range (**b**). Peripheral iridotomy was shown (*white arrow*). ROP = retinopathy of prematurity

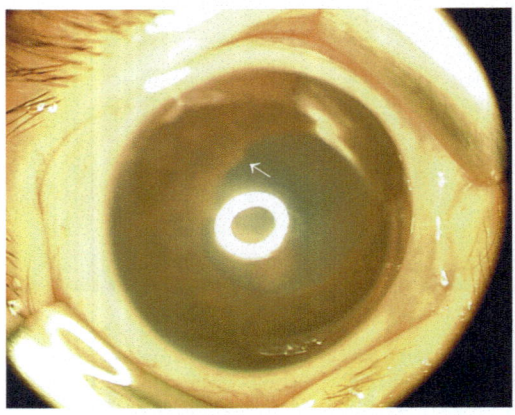

Fig. 11.10 Development of cataract 1 year after vitrectomy for stage 4 ROP. Posterior synechia was noted (*white arrow*). ROP = retinopathy of prematurity

operation is an extremely poor prognostic factor, with reattachment rate of 0% in the study by Lakhanpal et al. despite extensive membrane dissection, treatment of the retinal breaks, and the use of long-acting tamponade [36].

Before the operation, the fundus should be checked again to determine the configuration of the retinal detachment. The area with the least amount of retinal dragging is selected as the infusion site. This approach may reduce the incidence of an iatrogenic retinal tear. The vectors that involve tractional forces on the retina are dissected until the surgeon determines that the forces are relieved by the vitreous cutter [35]. Aggressive membrane peeling is avoided, and efforts are made to reduce the possibility of iatrogenic break, which usually carries with it a poor prognosis. Retinal flattening takes several months because of the exudative component in the subretinal space. Documentation of the surgical procedure is important and is performed using a video recording system.

Recently, Imaizumi et al. [37] advocated the short-term use of perfluoro-n-octane in complicated cases of ROP, such as cases with retinal breaks. The perfluoro-n-octane was removed after 1–4 weeks postoperatively. Perfluoro-n-octane has also been used in the case of complex pediatric retinal detachment with severe proliferative vitreoretinopathy (PVR) [38]. While the posterior proliferative changes are in the inferior retina and gas or silicone oil are considered less effective, perfluoro-n-octane can be considered as a temporary postoperative tamponade in complicated cases of ROP. Initial outcome is encouraging in these patients. Possible complications associated with vitrectomy are listed in Table 11.5, and Figs. 11.8, 11.9, 11.10 and 11.11.

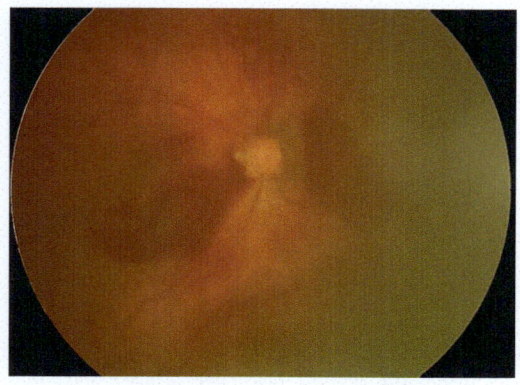

Fig. 11.11 Pre-retinal hemorrhage after vitrectomy in the right eye of a patient with stage 4 ROP. Pre-retinal hemorrhages usually reabsorb within weeks without treatment

References

1. Good WV. Final results of the early treatment for retinopathy of prematurity (ETROP) randomized trial. Trans Am Ophthalmol Soc. 2004;102:233–48.
2. Wu WC, Lin RI, Shih CP, et al. Visual acuity, optical components, and macular abnormalities in patients with a history of retinopathy of prematurity. Ophthalmol. 2012;119:1907–16.
3. Tasman W, Patz A, McNamara JA, et al. Retinopathy of prematurity: the life of a lifetime disease. Am J Ophthalmol. 2006;141:167–74.
4. Tufail A, Singh AJ, Haynes RJ, et al. Late onset vitreoretinal complications of regressed retinopathy of prematurity. Br J Ophthalmol. 2004;88:243–6.
5. Summers G, Phelps DL, Tung B, Palmer EA. Ocular cosmesis in retinopathy of prematurity. The cryotherapy for retinopathy of prematurity cooperative group. Arch Ophthalmol. 1992;110:1092–7.
6. Multicenter trial of cryotherapy for retinopathy of prematurity. Preliminary results. Cryotherapy for retinopathy of prematurity cooperative group. Arch Ophthalmol. 1988;106:471–9.
7. Multicenter trial of cryotherapy for retinopathy of prematurity. Three-month outcome. Cryotherapy for retinopathy of prematurity cooperative group. Arch Ophthalmol. 1990;108:195–204.
8. Multicenter trial of cryotherapy for retinopathy of prematurity. One-year outcome–structure and function. Cryotherapy for retinopathy of prematurity cooperative group. Arch Ophthalmol. 1990;108:1408–16.
9. Simpson JL, Melia M, Yang MB, et al. Current role of cryotherapy in retinopathy of prematurity: a report by the American academy of ophthalmology. Ophthalmol. 2012;119:873–7.
10. Jalali S, Azad R, Trehan HS, et al. Technical aspects of laser treatment for acute retinopathy of prematurity under topical anesthesia. Indian J Ophthalmol. 2010;58:509–15.
11. Sato T, Kusaka S, Shimojo H, Fujikado T. Simultaneous analyses of vitreous levels of 27 cytokines in eyes with retinopathy of prematurity. Ophthalmol. 2009.
12. Sato T, Kusaka S, Shimojo H, Fujikado T. Vitreous levels of erythropoietin and vascular endothelial growth factor in eyes with retinopathy of prematurity. Ophthalmol. 2009;116:1599–603.
13. Smith LE. Through the eyes of a child: understanding retinopathy through ROP the Friedenwald lecture. Invest Ophthalmol Vis Sci. 2008;49:5177–82.
14. Bakri SJ, Snyder MR, Reid JM, et al. Pharmacokinetics of intravitreal bevacizumab (Avastin). Ophthalmol. 2007;114:855–9.
15. Bakri SJ, Snyder MR, Reid JM, et al. Pharmacokinetics of intravitreal ranibizumab (Lucentis). Ophthalmol. 2007;114:2179–82.
16. Dorta P, Kychenthal A. Treatment of type 1 retinopathy of prematurity with intravitreal bevacizumab (Avastin). Retina. 2010;30:S24–31.
17. Lin CJ, Chen SN, Hwang JF. Intravitreal ranibizumab as salvage therapy in an extremely low-birth-weight infant with rush type retinopathy of prematurity. Oman J Ophthalmol. 2012;5:184–6.
18. Mintz-Hittner HA, Kennedy KA, Chuang AZ. Efficacy of intravitreal bevacizumab for stage 3 + retinopathy of prematurity. N Engl J Med. 2011;364:603–15.
19. Mota A, Carneiro A, Breda J, et al. Combination of intravitreal ranibizumab and laser photocoagulation for aggressive posterior retinopathy of prematurity. Case Rep Ophthalmol. 2012;3:136–41.
20. Castellanos MA, Schwartz S, Garcia-Aguirre G, Quiroz-Mercado H. Short-term outcome after intravitreal ranibizumab injections for the treatment of retinopathy of prematurity. Br J Ophthalmol. 2013;97:816–9.
21. Wu WC, Kuo HK, Yeh PT, et al. An updated study of the use of bevacizumab in the treatment of patients with prethreshold retinopathy of prematurity in Taiwan. Am J Ophthalmol. 2013;155:150–8.
22. Moshfeghi DM, Berrocal AM. Retinopathy of prematurity in the time of bevacizumab: incorporating the BEAT-ROP results into clinical practice. Ophthalmol. 2011;118:1227–8.
23. Sato T, Wada K, Arahori H, et al. Serum concentrations of bevacizumab (avastin) and vascular endothelial growth factor in infants with retinopathy of prematurity. Am J Ophthalmol. 2012;153:327–33.
24. Wu WC, Lai CC, Chen KJ, et al. Long-term tolerability and serum concentration of bevacizumab (avastin) when injected in newborn rabbit eyes. Invest Ophthalmol Vis Sci. 2010;51:3701–8.
25. Sakowski SA, Heavener SB, Lunn JS, et al. Neuroprotection using gene therapy to induce vascular

endothelial growth factor-A expression. Gene Ther. 2009;16:1292–9.

26. Been JV, Zoer B, Kloosterboer N, et al. Pulmonary vascular endothelial growth factor expression and disaturated phospholipid content in a chicken model of hypoxia-induced fetal growth restriction. Neonatology. 2010;97:183–9.

27. Yamamoto C, Yagi S, Hori T, et al. Significance of portal venous VEGF during liver regeneration after hepatectomy. J Surg Res. 2010;159:e37–43.

28. Martinez-Castellanos MA, Schwartz S, Hernandez-Rojas ML, et al. Long-term effect of antiangiogenic therapy for retinopathy of prematurity up to 5 years of follow-up. Retina. 2013;33:329–38.

29. Banker AS, Banker DA. Anatomical, functional, OCT and neurodevelopmental analysis outcomes of intravitreal bevacizumab injection without laser for retinopathy of prematurity: 6 year follow-up. 2013.

30. Micieli JA, Surkont M, Smith AF. A systematic analysis of the off-label use of bevacizumab for severe retinopathy of prematurity. Am J Ophthalmol. 2009;148:536–43.

31. Harder BC, Schlichtenbrede FC, von BS, et al. Intravitreal bevacizumab for retinopathy of prematurity: refractive error results. Am J Ophthalmol. 2013;155:1119–24.

32. Smith EL III. Prentice award lecture 2010: a case for peripheral optical treatment strategies for myopia. Optom Vis Sci. 2011;88:1029–44.

33. Chuang YC, Yang CM. Scleral buckling for stage 4 retinopathy of prematurity. Ophthalmic Surg Lasers. 2000;31:374–9.

34. Ricci B, Santo A, Ricci F, et al. Scleral buckling surgery in stage 4 retinopathy of prematurity. Graefes Arch Clin Exp Ophthalmol. 1996;234(Suppl 1):S38–41.

35. Wu WC, Lai CC, Lin RI, et al. Modified 23-gauge vitrectomy system for stage 4 retinopathy of prematurity. Arch Ophthalmol. 2011;129:1326–31.

36. Lakhanpal RR, Sun RL, Albini TA, Holz ER. Anatomical success rate after primary three-port lens-sparing vitrectomy in stage 5 retinopathy of prematurity. Retina. 2006;26:724–8.

37. Imaizumi A, Kusaka S, Noguchi H, et al. Efficacy of short-term postoperative perfluoro-n-octane tamponade for pediatric complex retinal detachment. Am J Ophthalmol. 2014;157:384–9.

38. Sisk RA, Berrocal AM, Murray TG, Mavrofrides EC. Extended endotamponade with perfluoro-n-octane in pediatric retinal detachment. Ophthalmic Surg Lasers Imaging. 2010;1–3.

Differential Diagnosis of ROP

George Caputo

Keywords

Retinal detachment · Retinopathy of prematurity (ROP) · Familial exudative vitreoretinopathy (FEVR) · Mutations · Exudation · Pediatric · Macular fold · Retinal ischemia

Retinopathy of prematurity can simulate a variety of conditions according to the stage of the disease.

The main characteristic of ROP is the development of extraretinal neovascular proliferation induced by large territories of non-perfused retina.

Differential diagnosis of ROP is not really an issue for early stages of the disease, the clinical features being specific. Advanced stages of ROP presenting with retinal detachment can be controversial and each clinical feature is seen in other diseases; retinal ischemia, subretinal exudation, retinal detachment, retinal dragging, retinal folds are observed in different congenital or evolving pediatric retinal diseases.

Medical History

The main answer to differential diagnosis of ROP is the past medical history of prematurity. The birth weight and term at risk for developing severe retinopathy of prematurity varies according to the country of birth, and is not the same in developed countries compared to developing regions. In Nepal, Babies less than 2000 g at birth and born at 36 WG or less have a 3.8% rate of stage 3 or more disease [1].

Genetic Background

Differential diagnosis of ROP concerns retinal diseases that share a common genetic background. Mutations in the NDP gene is a common feature present in Norrie disease shared with some cases of familial exudative vitreoretinopathy (FEVR) [2]. Norrin by its interaction with the product of FZD4 is implicated in the Wnt signaling pathway, crucial to angiogenesis. Mutations in FZD4, LRP5, TSPAN12, or ZNF408 genes are responsible for FEVR, and little phenotype genotype correlation has been established [3]. It has been reported in rare cases of Coat's disease and ROP a mutation in FZD4 gene [4]. Up to 3% of severe cases of ROP present mutations in the FZD4 gene that could explain surprising evolutions of the disease [5, 6].

Clinical Features

Retinal Ischemia

Famial Exudative Vitreoretinopathy

Peripheral retinal ischemia is a specific feature of ROP and is also observed in Familial exudative

G. Caputo (✉)
Department of Pediatric Ophthalmology, Rothschild Ophthalmological Foundation, 25 Rue Manin 75019 Paris, 75019 Paris, France
e-mail: gcaputo@fo-rothschild.fr

(a)   **(b)**

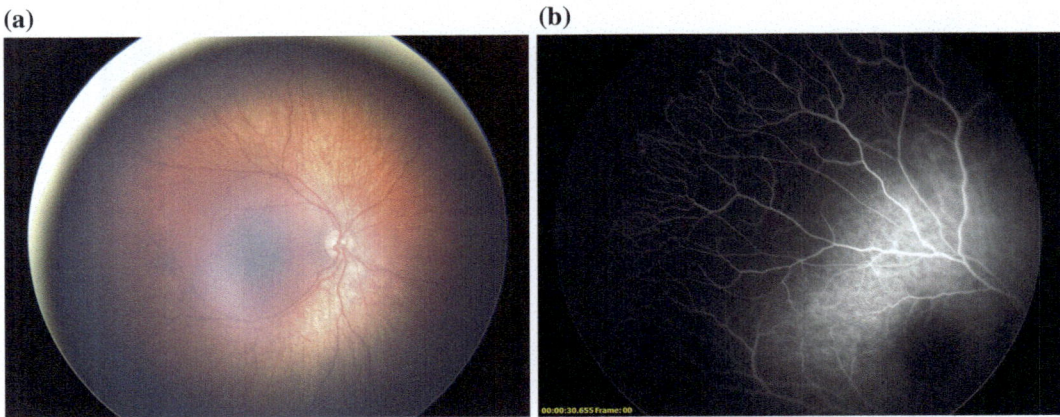

Fig. 12.1 Retinal ischemia in FEVR patient. Fundus photograph is unremarkable and wide angle angiography shows peripheral retinal ischemia

vitreoretinopathy (FEVR). In the latter, peripheral retinal ischemia develops during infancy inducing extraretinal neovascularization, leading in the late stages to tractional and exudative retinal detachment; ischemia predominates on the temporal retina, with thin peripheral vascular arborisation that ends with capillary drop-out (Fig. 12.1). FEVR is a genetic disease with dominant, recessive or X-linked transmission that develops with no history of prematurity. Mutations affect FRZL4, LRP5, Norrie, TSPAN12 or ZNF408 genes [7].

In advanced cases of FEVR with retinal detachment in young babies, the exudative component is often consistently present.

Incontinentia Pigmenti

Incontinentia pigmenti is a dominant genetic disease linked to chromosome X, lethal for boys. Retinal ischemia develops during the first year of life, and usually affects only one eye due to lionization of chromosome X (Fig. 12.2). Other specific features of this disease are the dermatological lesions that consist in pigmented skin lesions on the legs that are visible during the first months of life [8].

Shaken Baby Syndrome

We have described ischemic lesion in shaken baby syndrome that could be due to the shearing effect of the trauma on retinal vessels (Fig. 12.3) [9].

Subretinal Exudation

Subretinal exudation is less commonly seen in ROP, but can be observed in advanced stages of stage 4 or 5 disease with very active plus disease.

In FEVR, this feature can be predominant due to the presence of large vessel peripheral anastomosis.

Coats disease is characterized by vascular dilation of capillaries, rarefaction of capillary meshwork and retinal exudation leading to total retinal detachment (Figs. 12.4 and 12.5) [10]. Boys are specifically concerned in 85% of the cases. No vitreous involvement is observed initially in Coat's disease; neovascularization can be observed after induced retinal ischemia by extensive laser photocoagulation of vascular aneurysms [11].

Retinal Detachment

Retinal detachment is observed in stage 4 and 5 ROP. In late phases of these detachments, the fibrous tissue can be the predominant feature of these tractional detachments, with a very important regression of the vascular component in most cases.

Advanced stages of FEVR are characterized by total retinal detachment (Fig. 12.6). Although babies can be affected, the mean age of retinal

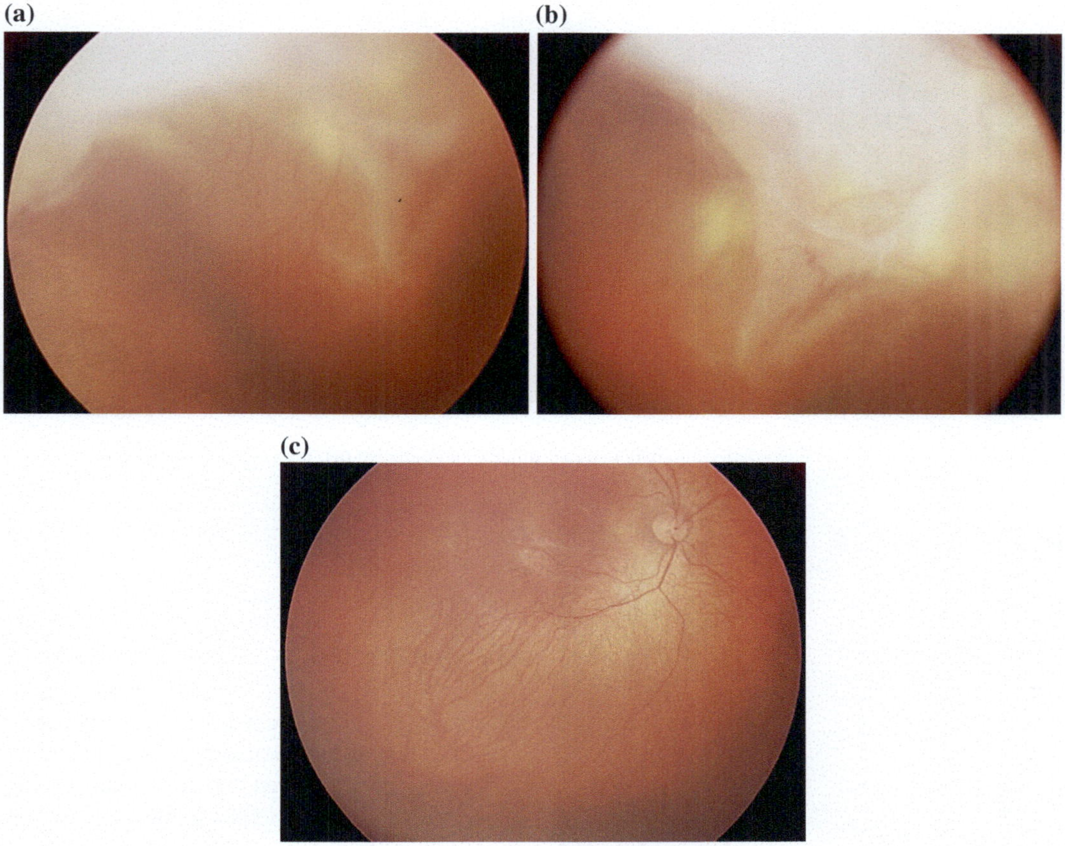

(a)   (b)

(c)

Fig. 12.2 Retinal ischemia and preretinal neovascularization in incontinentia pigmenti (**a**, **b**). Contralateral fundus photography showing mild vascular changes but inferior temporal ischemia

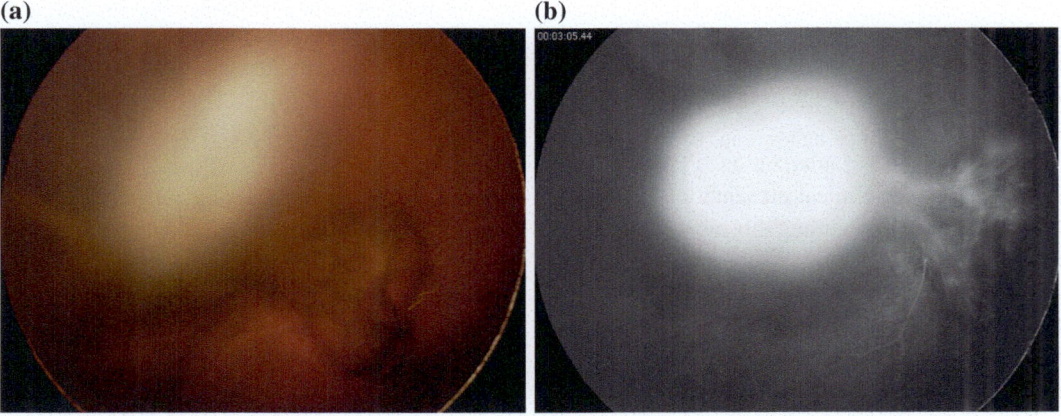

Fig. 12.3 Partial retinal detachment in a case of shaken baby syndrome: fundus photography (**a**), fluorescein angiogram showing extensive retinal ischemia (**b**)

(a) **(b)**

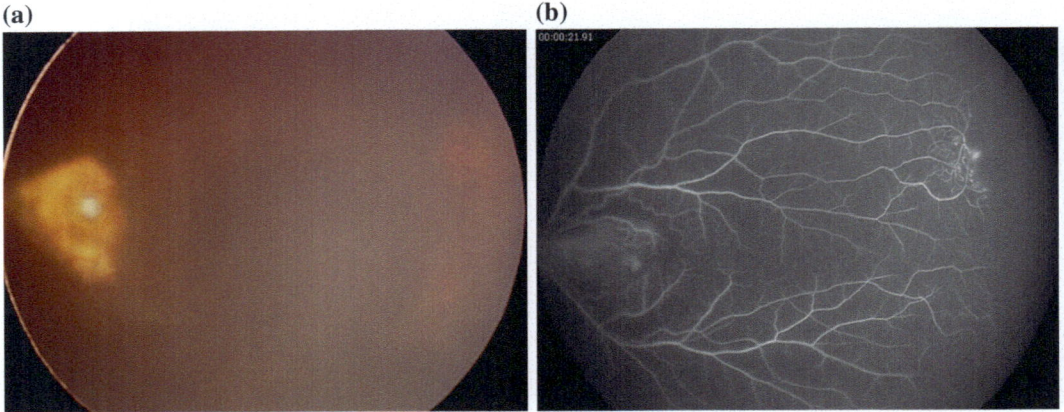

Fig. 12.4 Example of retinal exudation in coats disease, fundus retinography (**a**), fluorescein angiography (**b**)

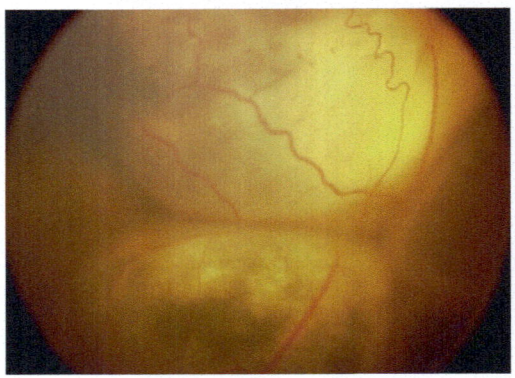

Fig. 12.5 A cases of retinal detachment due to coat's disease. *Note* The exudative nature of the detachment and the absence of vitreous involvement

detachment in this disease is young infancy or adolescence. Subretinal exudation is often present and asymmetrical disease is a typical presentation in FEVR.

Persistent fetal vascularization (PFV) can lead to a big variety of clinical presentation according to the degree of remaining fibrovascular tissue. Total retinal detachment is observed in severe cases, and the absence of vascular disease in the fellow eye can be the only way to confirm the diagnosis; wide angle angiography is recommended to eliminate peripheral retinal ischemia.

Retinal dysplasia is characterized by bilateral involvement of ocular lesions presenting the same clinical features as in PFV (Fig. 12.7) [12]. Norrie disease is an X-linked disease affecting

boys; hearing impairment and autistic disorder can be associated.

Macular Ectopia

Macular ectopia is the consequence of retinal dragging due to temporal extraretinal neovascularization and is shared by ROP and FEVR. A rectitude of the temporal vessels accompanies this ectopia.

Retinal Fold

Retinal folds are the cicatricial form of stage 4A and 4B ROP retinal detachments. Localized and progressive temporal fibrous tissue contraction leads to a macular fold. This feature can be observed in FEVR, PFV, Norrie disease, and retinal dysplasia [13] (Fig. 12.8).

The appearance of the retina outside the retinal fold brings significant information: the presence of vessels is more commonly seen in FEVR and ROP (the absence of vessels and heavy epiretinal alterations are more commonly encountered in PFV and retinal dysplasia (Fig. 12.9).

In summary, differential diagnosis of ROP is easy in the presence of a typical medical history; it can be tricky when some degree of prematurity is present according to the standards of care in the country of origin. Many diseases can simulate

(a)

(b)

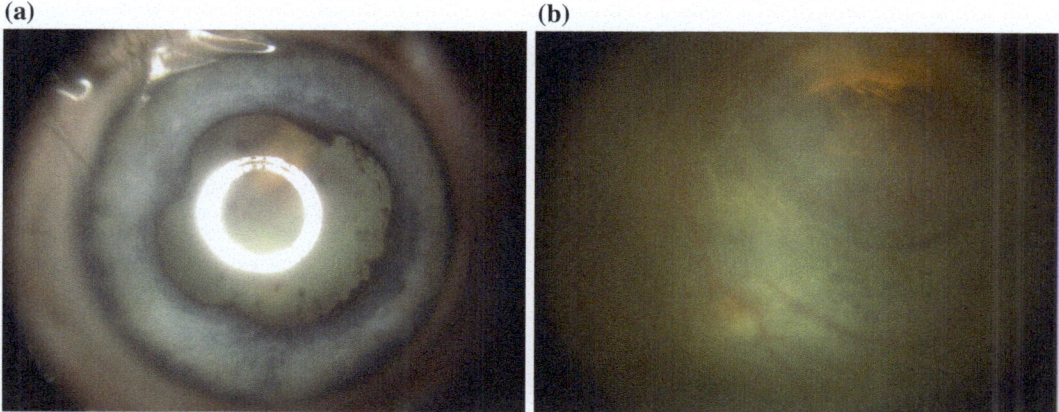

Fig. 12.6 A case of unilateral total retinal detachment in FEVR comparable to stage 5 ROP

(a)

(b)

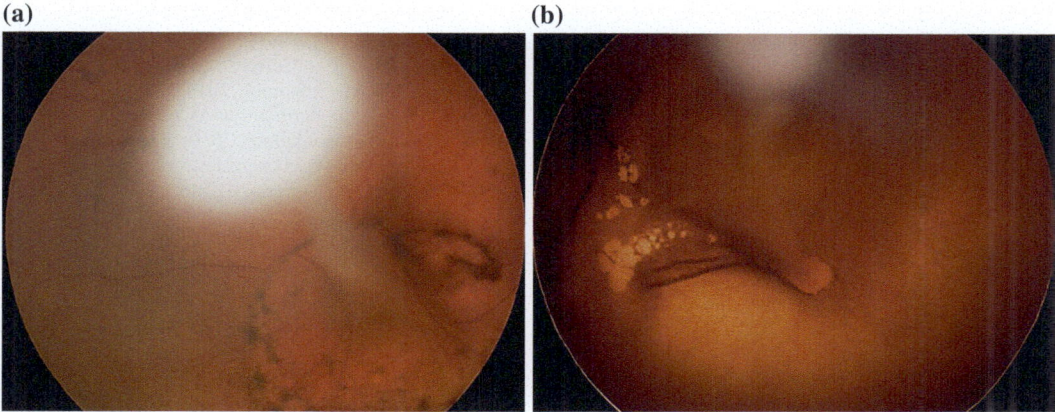

Fig. 12.7 Retinal dysplasia responsible for bilateral retinal fold. *Note* The pigmentary subretinal changes that help recognizing diagnosis

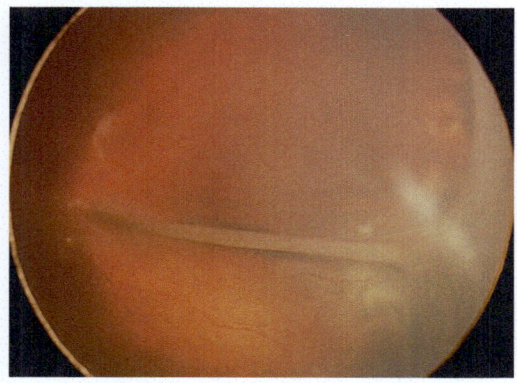

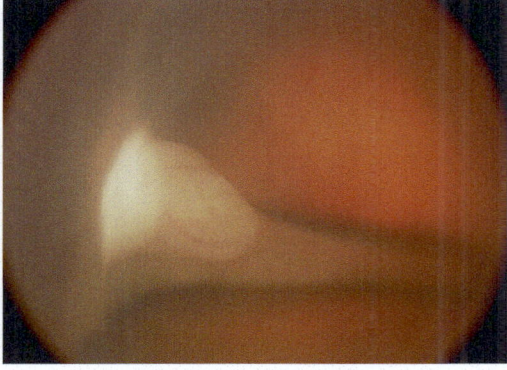

Fig. 12.8 A case of unilateral retinal fold in FEVR *Note* The exudates and extraretinal neovascularization

Fig. 12.9 Unilateral retinal fold due to persistent featal vascularization

specific clinical features of ROP, and a thorough analysis of the observed lesions helped by wide-angle angiography allows leading to the right diagnosis. All these differential diagnosis of ROP share some common genetic interactions with the Norrie/FZD4 Wnt signaling pathway implicated in angiogenesis and the comprehension and analysis of these mechanisms will help us in diagnosis and classification of the diseases.

References

1. Shrestha JB, et al. Incidence of retinopathy of prematurity in a neonatal intensive care unit in Nepal. J Pediatr Ophthalmol Strabismus. 2010;47 (5):297–300.
2. Dickinson JL, et al. Mutations in the NDP gene: contribution to Norrie disease, familial exudative vitreoretinopathy and retinopathy of prematurity. Clin Experiment Ophthalmol. 2006;34(7):682–8.
3. Wu WC, et al. Retinal phenotype-genotype correlation of pediatric patients expressing mutations in the Norrie disease gene. Arch Ophthalmol. 2007;125 (2):225–30.
4. Drenser KA, et al. Clinical presentation and genetic correlation of patients with mutations affecting the FZD4 gene. Arch Ophthalmol. 2009;127(12):1649–54.
5. Shastry BS, et al. Identification of missense mutations in the Norrie disease gene associated with advanced retinopathy of prematurity. Arch Ophthalmol. 1997;115(5):651–5.
6. Ells A, et al. Severe retinopathy of prematurity associated with FZD4 mutations. Ophthalmic Genet. 2010;31(1):37–43.
7. Gilmour DF. Familial exudative vitreoretinopathy and related retinopathies. Eye (Lond). 2015;29(1):1–14.
8. Holmstrom G, Thoren K. Ocular manifestations of incontinentia pigmenti. Acta Ophthalmol Scand. 2000;78(3):348–53.
9. Caputo G, et al. Ischemic retinopathy and neovascular proliferation secondary to shaken baby syndrome. Retina. 2008;28(3 Suppl):S42–6.
10. Morris B, Foot B, Mulvihill A. A population-based study of Coats disease in the United Kingdom I: epidemiology and clinical features at diagnosis. Eye (Lond). 2010;24(12):1797–801.
11. Sigler EJ, et al. Current management of Coats disease. Surv Ophthalmol. 2014;59(1):30–46.
12. Walsh MK, et al. Early vitrectomy effective for Norrie disease. Arch Ophthalmol. 2010;128(4):456–60.
13. Nishina, S., et al., Clinical features of congenital retinal folds. Am J Ophthalmol. 2012;153(1): p. 81–7.

Anesthesia for Preterms with Retinopathy of Prematurity

13

María Eliana Eberhard and Patricio A. Leyton

Keywords

Anesthesia for new born · Retinopathy of prematurity (ROP) · Sevoflurane · Airway management · Ventilation · Inhalational anesthesia

Retinopathy of the newborn (ROP) is the most frequent ocular pathology in preterm infants. Standard pediatric anesthesia works well in older infant and children undergoing ophthalmologic surgery. However, anesthesia may be extremely complex and delicate in acutely ill preterm infants, very low birth weight infants, or those younger than 1 year of age afflicted with ROP. These patients are at greater risk than older children and demand a special care when general anesthesia is needed, almost always requiring an experienced pediatric anesthesiologist.

The preterm infant may have significant systemic illnesses. Common complications of prematurity include, among others, acute and chronic pulmonary diseases, respiratory failure and pulmonary hypertension, congenital heart disease, and intraventricular cerebral hemorrhage. Two main issues arise from anesthetizing preterm infants with ROP: airway management and apnea.

Airway Management

Careful attention to airway management, assisted ventilation, and titration of oxygen therapy with specified goals are essential for success. In mechanically ventilated preterm infants, the anesthesiologist should confirm the position of the tube, transport the infant safely to the operating room, and limit the exposure to high concentration of oxygen. Attention should be taken not to develop hypercarbia and hypoxia, occurring commonly as a result of apnea and hypoventilation during emergency and recovery from anesthesia, since both can lead to increase in choroidal blood volume and intraocular pressure [11].

Apnea

Perioperative apnea in preterm infant is widely described and can occur in 7% of neonates born at 34–35 weeks gestation, 15% at 32–33 weeks, more than 50% at 30–31 weeks, and as high as almost 100% of micropremie (less than 1000 kg)

M.E. Eberhard (✉)
Anesthesia and Pain Unit, Universidad Del Desarollo, Clinica Alemana de Santiago, Lo Gallo 2272 Vitacura, 7640177 Santiago, Region Metropolitana, Chile
e-mail: eberhard.maria.eliana@gmail.com

P.A. Leyton
Anestesiología, Clínica Alemana de Santiago, Avenida Vitacura 5951 Vitacura, 7650568 Santiago, Región Metropolitana, Chile
e-mail: pleyton@gmail.com

© Springer International Publishing AG 2017
Andrés Kychenthal B. and Paola Dorta S. (eds.), *Retinopathy of Prematurity*,
DOI 10.1007/978-3-319-52190-9_13

[14]. Preoperative assessment should determine in advance the occurrence, pattern, and frequency of apnea. Those factors should be considered whether the child is still an inpatient or an outpatient. Should the child be discharged, the current use of respiratory stimulants, oxygen, and/or the use or continuation of an apnea monitor must be determined. Perioperative apnea may preclude tracheal extubation or require close postoperative monitoring after anesthesia [10].

Temperature Management

Preterm and small infants rapidly loose heat when anesthetized. Therefore, prevention of hypothermia is essential in the perioperative environment. Hypothermia can decrease metabolism of most drugs and depresses respiratory drive in preterm infants. Additionally, infants with extremely low birth weight require many weeks to grow and develop to a weight of approximately 1800 g and to maintain normothermia without special environmental control [8]. Apnea may also be a complication of hypothermia, leading to unnecessary postprocedural mechanical ventilation, exposing the patient to new complications or to worsen previous basal cerebral and pulmonary conditions.

Other Considerations

Preoperative assessment should also include the child's developmental and neurologic status at the time of surgery. Intraventricular cerebral hemorrhage (IVH) complicates preterm infants frequently. Mechanically ventilation is one of the risk factors to develop IVH in preterm infants. Anesthesia in those preterm infants not infrequently requires postoperative mechanical ventilation.

To prevent and treat possible complications, intravenous access should be always obtained in advance of the surgical procedure or any examination.

Anesthesia Management

An ophthalmologic examination under anesthesia is essential for an accurate diagnosis as well for evaluations of the progress of ROP and the response of the disease to treatment. Ophthalmologic examinations and procedures may be performed in the neonatal care unit or in the operating room and may require sedation or general anesthesia. For surgical ROP therapy, infants require general anesthesia to provide optimal surgical conditions.

Many different technical approaches can be used [2, 5, 9]. Sevoflurane is the most commonly inhalational anesthetic agent used for pediatric patients. Sevoflurane provides a rapid induction and emergence from general anesthesia. Respiratory support during and following examinations, laser surgery or intravitreal injection of antiangiogenic agents is commonly accomplished using endotracheal intubation and mechanical ventilation. Frequently, newborns undergoing ophtalmological treatments or ROP surgery have been weaned off mechanical ventilation days or weeks before the procedure. When they are electively re-intubated for ROP treatment, postoperative extubation can be cumbersome and may require prolonged ventilatory support. Avoidance of tracheal intubation for short procedure would be the best way to keep the newborn out of mechanical ventilation [13].

Laser therapy, cryotherapy, and currently the intravitreal injection of antiangiogenic agents are the most common treatments for ROP. Because of the accuracy required to perform the procedure, an immobile field is necessary. In some cases, it is recommendable tracheal intubation with neuromuscular relaxants, providing better perioperative stability for the newborn [4]. Nevertheless, in an attempt to avoid intubation and mechanical ventilation, and their complications, we consider another approach to provide general anesthesia with inhaled agents. This technique consists in administering inhaled anesthetic agents through a nasal cannula with an in-made sideline to monitor end tidal CO_2. The nasal nostrils with the cannula in place are then sealed with a tape to provide continuous airflow. In our experience, it is an alternative way to keep a continuous positive airway pressure during general anesthesia without tracheal intubation [1, 3, 7].

Prematurity with its wide spectrum of clinical presentation and complications determines the most adequate anesthesia technique [6]. In general, premature babies need a warm perioperative environment to reduce thermal stress. To determine whether sedation or general anesthesia provided with endotracheal tube, laryngeal mask, or nasal cannula is the most appropriate technique, the clinical experience of the anesthesiologist and the hospital center support has to be taken into account. For example, adequate support and monitoring for postoperative period with babies that require ventilator supporting an intensive neonatal care unit [12].

References

1. Azar P, Dimister A, Visas N. Recomendaciones para uso de CPAP en recien nacido de pretermino. Archivos Argentinos de Pediatria. 2001;99(5):451–5.
2. Chen SD, Sundaram V, Wilkinson A, Patel CK. Variation in anaesthesia for the laser treatment of retinopathy of prematurity—a survey of ophthalmologists in the UK. Eye. 2007;21(8):1033–6. doi:10.1038/sj.eye.6702499.
3. Eberhard M. Anestesia general ambulatoria en recien nacidos prematuris con retinopatia. Revista Chilena de Anestesia. 2008;37(3):202.
4. Eberhard M, Kychenthal A, Dorta P, Alvarez M. Anestesia general para prematuros con retinopatia y alta antes de las 36 semanas. Revista Chilena de Anestesia. 2004;33:229–30.
5. Haigh PM, Chiswick ML, O'Donoghue EP. Retinopathy of prematurity: systemic complications associated with different anaesthetic techniques at treatment. Br J Ophthalmol. 1997;81(4):283–7.
6. Hartrey R. Anaesthesia for the laser treatment of neonates with retinopathy of prematurity. Eye. 2007;21(8):1025–7. doi:10.1038/sj.eye.6702502.
7. Higgins RD, Richter SE, Davis JM. Nasal continuous positive airway pressure facilitates extubation of very low birth weight neonates. Pediatrics. 1991;88 (5):999–1003.
8. Jahnukainen T, van Ravenswaaij-Arts C, Jalonen J, Valimaki I. Dynamics of vasomotor thermoregulation of the skin in term and preterm neonates. Early Hum Dev. 1993;33(2):133–43.
9. Lyon F, Dabbs T, O'Meara M. Anaesthesia in retinopathy of prematurity treatment. Eye. 2008;22 (1):165. doi:10.1038/sj.eye.6703048.
10. Peiris K, Fell D. The prematurely born infant and anaesthesia. Cont Edu Anaesth, Crit Care Pain. 2009;9(3):73–7. doi:10.1093/bjaceaccp/mkp010.
11. Wangsa-Wirawan ND, Linsenmeier RA. Retinal oxygen: fundamental and clinical aspects. Arch Ophthalmol. 2003;121(4):547–57. doi:10.1001/archopht.121.4.547.
12. Welborn LG, Greenspun JC. Anesthesia and apnea. perioperative considerations in the former preterm infant. Pediatr Clin North Am. 1994;41(1):181–98.
13. Woodhead DD, Lambert DK, Molloy DA, Schmutz N, Righter E, Baer VL, Christensen RD. Avoiding endotracheal intubation of neonates undergoing laser surgery for retinopathy of prematurity. J Perinatol: Off J Calif Perinat Assoc. 2007;27 (4):209–13. doi:10.1038/sj.jp.7211675.
14. Zhao J, Gonzalez F, Mu D. Apnea of prematurity: from cause to treatment. Eur J Pediatr. 2011;170 (9):1097–105. doi:10.1007/s00431-011-1409-6.

Neonatologist Perspectives on ROP

14

Monica Morgues

Abstract

Because neonatologists have achieved better results in the survival of premature children, neurosensory complications have increased, including retinopathy of prematurity (ROP). The main goals are the prevention and monitoring of a timely diagnosis. It is thus necessary to prevent premature births, apply adequate therapeutic management in the NICU, and avoid exposure to factors that increase the risk of ROP. Pathophysiological studies have helped us to learn how the immature retina develops in the extra-uterine environment to optimize prevention and to develop new therapies that cause less damage when applied. Supporting ophthalmologists in all interventions leads to improved diagnosis, particularly when expertise is required, even when retina specialist is not available, using digital technologies. Neonatologists should focus on optimizing neonatal intensive care management and ensure that the child and family screening is adequate, timely, and performed by an expert.

Keywords

Retinopathy of prematurity (ROP) · Premature birth · Visually impaired children · Postnatal care · Hyperoxia · Intrauterine grow retardation

Introduction

Retinopathy of prematurity (ROP) is a vascular proliferative disease that affects normal retinal development in premature newborns. There is detention in the vascular growth and then an abnormal maturation of vessels. If the disease is severe, it can lead to permanent ocular damage, retinal detachment, and blindness.

M. Morgues (✉)
Pediatric Department, Campus North, Universidad de Chile/San José Hospital, Zañuartu 1085
Independencia, 7710087 Santiago, Chile
e-mail: mimorgues@gmail.com

© Springer International Publishing AG 2017
Andrés Kychenthal B. and Paola Dorta S. (eds.), *Retinopathy of Prematurity*,
DOI 10.1007/978-3-319-52190-9_14

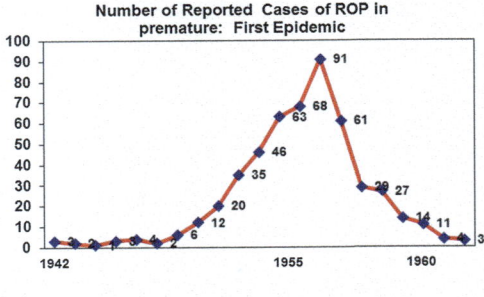

Number of Reported Cases of ROP in
premature: First Epidemic

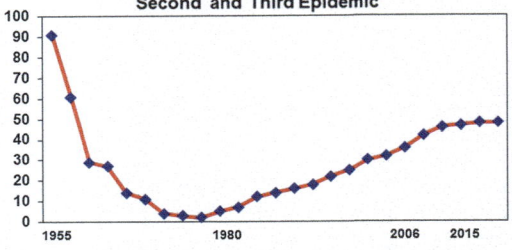

Second and Third Epidemic

Fig. 14.1 Number of reported cases of ROP in premature. **a** First epidemic; **b** second and third epidemics

The neonatal disease perspective of ROP has
focused on prevention and therapy that should be
adequate and timely and should cause fewer side
effects. This sentence seems so simple to write,
but it encompasses all of the problems faced by
neonatology in the history of the disease that
have not yet been fully resolved.

Since it was first described by Theodore Terry
in 1942 [1] and then in 1951, was related to the
administration of oxygen in preterm infants with
respiratory disease, the focus has evolved through
periods of restriction of oxygen to stop what is
known as the first epidemic of ROP, which
occurred in the 1950s, when there was a dramatic
decrease in cases, but a serious increase in

cerebral palsy in premature infants over the next
decade [2]. The impact of these events has generated a different practice, based on evidence and
moderation of oxygen therapy in neonatal units;
as a result, the disease has appeared again, but
with a higher incidence in children with fewer
weeks of gestation at birth. This second epidemic
has produced many studies and evidence, and in
particular, the technological progress has also
been impressive. Many immature infants now
survive, maintaining a high incidence of ROP in
very immature preterm infants. When this technology reached developing countries, it increased
the number of surviving very immature infants,
thus starting what has been called the third epidemic of ROP (Fig. 14.1).

The WHO has estimated that there are 19 million visually impaired children, 1.4 million of
whom are blind. Its incidence is between 0.2 and
7.8/10,000 children, depending on the mortality
rates of children younger than 5 years old, based
on data that are available from each region and
country. In industrialized countries such as the
UK, [3] which recently published a comprehensive study on the subject, it was noted that cases
doubled from 0.17 to 0.41/10,000 children by the
age of 15 years old [4]. Cataracts, diabetic
retinopathy, glaucoma, and ROP are the major
causes of childhood blindness and visual impairment (Table 14.1) [5], and they are among the
priorities of the Pan American Health Organization (PAHO). The Action Plan on Eye
Health VISION 2020 Latin America was officially
launched in 2004 as a partnership among PAHO,
the Pan American Association of Ophthalmology
(PAAO), Initiatives for Blind Prevention of the

Table 14.1 The different causes of childhood severe visual impairment/ blindness	Causes by anatomical site	%
	Cerebral visual pathways	40
	Retina	24
	Optic nerve	23
	Whole globe and anterior ocular segment	6
	Cornea/Lens/Uvea	3
	Glaucoma	2
	Other	2

Adapted by permission from BMJ Publishing Group Limited [3], copyright 2014

Table 14.2 Preterm birth
rates by country

Country	Preterm birth/100 livebirths
Latvia	5.3
Croatia	5.5
Finland	5.5
Lithuania	5.7
Estonia	5.7
Japan	5.9
Sweden	5.9
Norway	6.0
Slovakia	6.3
Ireland	6.4
Italy	6.5
Greece	6.6
Denmark	6.7
France	6.7
Poland	6.7
Chile	7.1
Czech Republic	7.3
Switzerland	7.4
Spain	7.4
Slovenia	7.5
New Zealand	7.6
United Arab Emirates	7.6
Australia	7.6
Portugal	7.7
Argentina	8.0
Israel	8.0
Germany	9.2
Austria	10.9
USA	12.0
Costa Rica	13.6
Ghana	14.5
Cyprus	14.7
Pakistan	15.8
Mozambique	16.4
Zimbabwe	16.6
Congo	16.6
Malawi	18.1

See Ref. [13]

WHO, and nongovernmental organizations such as VISION 2020 "Right to Sight", and it has made changes to the work of health systems and the development of national plans for children in many countries [6]. The strategies of vitamin A supplementation and measles immunization have increased coverage, and the blindness from these causes has been eliminated in many developing countries [7]. ROP is now the foremost problem, especially in most industrializing countries in Latin America and Asia, where the survival of VLBW infants has improved considerably over the last decade. Cases are concentrated in less developed countries that have a higher incidence of prematurity (Table 14.2).

Perinatal Strategies in the Prevention of ROP

Neonatologists should focus their work in ROP on various strategies applied at different times in clinical practice.

Prenatal Care

Fetuses grow and develop in a relatively hypoxic environment, but with sufficient oxygen (O_2) to meet their needs. If available oxygen decreases, the fetus has specifics mechanisms of adaptation and compensation. The fetal arterial O_2 pressure is close to 20–25 mm Hg. This low pressure is "misleading", and oxygen availability during stress depends on the amount of oxygen delivery with blood perfusion (systemic oxygen transport) and tissue requirements (oxygen demand) and not only oxygen stress. Fetal hemoglobin (Hb F) provides the fetus with the ability to carry more oxygen from the placenta. It requires more oxygen than adult hemoglobin in the same concentrations, which allows it to absorb oxygen placental hemoglobin, with an oxygen pressure less than that in the maternal lung.

Prevention of preterm birth should be a joint effort with the obstetric team [8], sensitizing doctors to the impact of prematurity on the visual health of children and optimizing interventions in pregnant women. The use of antenatal steroids has small protective effects, so steroids should work to improve coverage of those at risk for preterm birth [9].

It has been postulated that vascular development and angiogenesis are the results of complex interactions between growth factors and mitogens, both locally and systemically produced, which stimulate or inhibit cell differentiation, proliferation, migration, and maturation of endothelial cells. Hellstrom et al. reported that low levels of insulin-like growth factor (IGF-I) in preterm patients were associated with ROP; in addition, these levels are as good a predictor of the disease as gestational age and birth weight. Recently, IGF levels were associated with ROP by intraocular quantification, varying with repeated fluctuations between hyperoxia and hypoxia [10]. This finding suggests that these cytokines might increase understanding of the observed clinical findings after these fluctuations in ROP. The regulation of the expression of vascular endothelial growth factor (VEGF) and other cytokines can contribute both to normal retinal vascular growth and to abnormal disruption and subsequent neovascularization. VEGF gene expression is regulated by many factors, including hypoxia, which is a potent inducer of VEGF by increasing gene transcription and stability in RNA, growth factors, cytokines, and other extracellular molecules [11, 12].

Perinatal Strategies to Be Implemented (Table 14.3) [13]

Surveillance of risk factors for preterm birth and controlling them.

Screening for urinary tract infections of pregnant women.

Treatment of bacterial vaginal infections.

Surveillance of twin pregnancies.

Length measurement of the uterine cervix at 20–22 weeks of gestation; if less than 25 mm in longitude, it is associated with a 40% rate of preterm birth.

Table 14.3 Contribution of risk factors to extremely, very, and moderately preterm births—register-based analysis of 1,390,742 singleton births

Adjusted odds ratio by risk factor	Extremely preterm OR (IC)	Very preterm OR (IC)
Maternal age: 30–39 (years)	1.25 (1.16–1.36)	1.24 (1.17–1.33)
Pregravid BMI ≥ 30	1.48 (1.20–1.82)	1.46 (1.24–1.74)
Smoking	1.21 (1.09–1.34)	1.23 (1,33–1.34)
Not married or cohabiting	1.31 (1.12–1.54)	1.32 (1.16–1.50)
Prior miscarriages	1.41 (1.36–1.46)	1.26 (1.22–1.31)
In vitro fertilization	2.14 (1.63–2.82)	1.52 (1.18–1.96)
Anemia ≤ 100 g/l	2.48 (1.82–3.38)	1.48 (1.08–2.04)
Chorionic villus biopsy	1.80 (1.38–2.33)	1.20 (0.93–1.56)
Amniocentesis	2.04 (1.75–2.37)	1.58 (1.38–1.82)
SGA	7.35 (6.69–8.09)	7.93 (7.35–8.55)
Mayor congenital anomaly	3.57 (3.17–4.01)	4.70 (4.31–5.12)
Stillbirth	4.46 (3.68–5.42)	3.73 (3.10–4.49)

Adjusted odds ratios (a ORs) of singleton extremely preterm and very preterm births for the years 1987–2010 in Finland [8]

Uterine artery Doppler ultrasound at 22–24 weeks to identify the risk of changes due to preeclampsia.

Treatment with progesterone or cervical cerclage perhaps indicated.

Use of tocolytics to delay delivery in cases of early labor.

Use of antenatal steroids.

Postnatal Care

Advances in the Neonatological Treatment of Prematurity, the "Better Practices"

The principal risk factors described are prematurity, oxygen therapy, male sex, and white race. Other risk factors have also been identified: delays in pre- and postnatal growth, assisted ventilation for more than 1 week, surfactant therapy, high volume blood transfusions, the use of erythropoietin and severe disease have been independently associated with higher rates of ROP.

The key is the prevention of ROP, for which we should emphasize the importance of identifying and reducing known risk factors.

Oxygen as a Principal Risk Factor

Oxygen is essential for cell functioning. The fetus develops normally in a hypoxic environment, and mechanisms to neutralize the adverse effects of high levels of oxygen are not fully developed. The range of oxygen and its requirements are not known and are variable during fetal development. Oxygen plays an important role in the pathogenesis of ROP; both hypoxia and hyperoxia will trigger a cascade of events that can lead to retinopathy [2, 14, 15]. Longer and uncontrolled high inspiration of oxygen concentration therapy severely increases the risk of ROP.

Excess oxygen interrupts normal vascular development and starts stimuli that can lead to ROP [16]. The retina is rich in polyunsaturated fatty acids, and it can easily produce lipid peroxidation and free radicals. Prostaglandin generation plays an important role in the regulation of ocular blood flow. Nitric oxide is very active in the choroid coat of the globe of the newborn, and it also regulates local flow. Interaction between increased PaO_2 and the perfusion pressure in the retina causes hyperoxia and initiates vascular alterations with the aberrant vessel characteristics of ROP. The most cost-effective action in the prevention of ROP is the prevention of preterm birth and rational and controlled use of oxygen [17].

Cautious administration of oxygen should be considered in three periods in premature infants: immediately after birth; during the acute phase of respiratory illness and recovery of neonatal distress; and at the time when bronchopulmonary dysplasia (BPD) begins.

After birth, many premature infants require supplemental oxygen to achieve adequate levels of oxygenation in the first 20 min of life. In the resuscitation of preterm infants <32 weeks old, an initial oxygen concentration between 30 and 40% is appropriate to reach saturation of 80–85% at 5 min of life and to stabilize at 88–92% at 20 min [18].

Early in the acute stages of illness, oxygen-saturation targets should be maintained at a low range of 88–92% to reduce the risk of ROP. Pulse oximetry is the best method to measure O_2 saturation (SpO_2) [19]. The correlation between SpO_2 and PaO_2 can be difficult to interpret because the affinity of fetal Hb to oxygen can be affected under different physiological conditions. Castillo et al. showed in preterm infants that SpO_2 values between 85 and 93% were correlated well with a mean PaO_2 of 56 ± 14.7 mm Hg, whereas SpO_2 was 93%, and PaO_2 increased to 107.3 ± 59.3. SpO_2 limits must be maintained in the prescribed range. Surfactant use in RDS allows for less use of O_2 in quantity and duration (Table 14.4).

The incidence of BPD increase when high SpO_2 values are used during the recovery period, and more frequent hospitalizations for respiratory diseases during early childhood have been seen, as evidenced in the BOOST study. Present evidence suggests that it is unwise to target oxygen-saturation values less than 90% in preterm infants born before 28 weeks of gestation. In the STOP-ROP study, 48% of infants on conventional oxygen (target 89–95%) and 41% of infants on supplemental oxygen (target 96–99%) progressed to threshold ROP. After adjustment for baseline factors, there was no significant difference between the groups. However, the supplemental oxygen group had worse systemic outcomes, with pneumonia or worsening chronic lung disease in 13.2%, compared to 8.5% in the conventional oxygen group. The monitoring of SpO2 should maintain the range in the appropriate range of SpO2 90–94% [20–22].

ROP Screening and Treatment

Early detection and timely treatment allow for better therapeutic performance [23–25]. Preterm infants that should be monitored according to the international guidelines for ROP prevention include babies with gestational ages equal to or less than 32 weeks with birth weights equal to or less than 1500 g, as well as those with birth weights greater than 1500 g and/or >32 weeks of gestational age who received oxygen for periods longer than 72 h. Risk factors that should be monitored in ROP include the following:

Newborns at Risk

1. Mechanical respiratory assistance
2. Prolonged or poorly monitored oxygen
3. IVH III–IV
4. DAP
5. DBP

Table 14.4 Summary meta-analysis of severe ROP in infants in low versus high oxygen-saturation target

Study	Relative risk (95% IC)
Support	0.52 (0.37–0.73)
BOOST (UK)	0.79 (0.60–1.06)
BOOST (AU)	0.76 (0.49–1.18)
BOOST (NZ)	0.86 (0.39–1.89)
COT	0.95 (0.65–1.39)
Overall	0.74 (0.59–0.92)

RRs and 95% IC's are given. RR exceeding 1 favors a high oxygen-saturation target

6. Another chronic illness requiring O_2
7. Transfusions of blood
8. Hyperoxia, hypoxia, or hypercapnia–hypocapnea
9. Shock
10. Apnea
11. Resuscitation techniques
12. Moderate to severe acidosis
13. Sepsis
14. Multiple gestations
15. Malnutrition
16. Deficiency in vitamin E

Intrauterine grow retardation (IUGR) and postnatal malnutrition have been reported to be important risk factors associated with ROP [7]. Infants who are small for their gestational age and below the 10th percentile should be considered at increased risk for developing prethreshold ROP versus AGA without grow restriction ($p < 0.01$), and they were more likely to develop severe ROP [26].

Administration of **erythropoietin** (rhEPO) reduces the need for transfusions, but it has been linked to a higher incidence and more severe course of ROP. It is a glycoprotein that stimulates the proliferation and differentiation of precursors of red blood cells, and it also affects the migration and proliferation of endothelial cells in retinal neovascularization processes, thus promoting angiogenesis. Both in vitro and in vivo, it exhibits the same angiogenic potential in endothelial cells, such as VEGF [27]. RhEPO is present in the development of the human retina, particularly in the region of activated mitosis. In the study by Kevin et al., rhEPO administration was an independent risk factor for ROP. Brown et al. reported that early administration of rhEPO was associated with an increased risk of ROP (OR 1.27). ROP was increased when rhEPO was administered within the 3 weeks after birth or during the first 8 days of life to prevent anemia; therefore, rhEPO is not recommended in preterm infants [28].

Infections can worsen the course of ROP [29]. In a study of children with ROP, those with positive Candida blood cultures were more likely to reach the threshold for ROP requiring surgery (OR 7.4, 95% CI 1.7–32.1). The infection was also associated with a poor outcome after laser photocoagulation.

Nutritional The risk of developing ROP also appears to be related to difficulties in increasing weight and size and to serum levels of IGF-1 and IGFBP-3 [30]. Postnatal weight predicts the occurrence of ROP at the sixth week of life. Weight gain <50% of newborn weight at the sixth week of life is a risk factor for developing ROP [31, 32]. Anemia aggravates the outcomes of ROP, particularly in the first 28 days of life. The visual system has strict nutritional requirements for the appropriate development of the photoreceptors and membrane cells in the visual cortex [12]. In both, more than 60% of the structures are formed by lipids with high concentrations of docosahexaenoic acid. Preterm birth incurs a high risk of deficiency of this fatty acid if it is not provided in the diet because precursor fatty acids production is limited [33]. Children not supplemented with diets rich in docosahexaenoic acid showed deficits in visual function.

Surfactants act as a protective factor decreasing the incidence of ROP due to decreased time and duration of oxygen therapy [34].

Transfusions Hb F (fetal) has a higher affinity for oxygen than adult Hb, so transfusions of red blood cells from adult donors increase free blood oxygen, and they increase the risk of ROP [27].

Phototherapy and light It was shown that there is a relationship between luminous therapy and disease progression. The study published by J.D. Reynolds in 1998 showed that there was no impact in preventing ROP of reduced exposure to light. Light is no longer considered to be a risk factor [35].

Carbon dioxide The vasodilatory action of carbon dioxide increases the area of the endothelium exposed to the toxic action of oxygen. Some studies have found a direct relationship between ROP and hypercapnia [36].

Different NICUs have different neonatal practices and experiences, so the risk of ROP varies among them. General ophthalmologists are responsible for surveillance and early diagnosis of ROP, but Type-1 retinopathy requires immediate therapeutic and diagnostic approaches, and expertise is necessary because a child who is blind from birth involves deep and costly limitations for the rest of his or her life. European countries have estimated this cost at € 300,000 over 50 years of life without considering educational costs [37–39]. A child with neurodevelopment limitations causes enormous disturbances of family relationships [40]. Ophthalmologist has used telemedicine diagnosis with digital images of the retina to solve this problem. Now it is possible to coordinate remote diagnostics with ophthalmologists who are experts in ROP. Telemedicine has successfully reduced late surgical intervention, improving visual prognosis. Photos constitute important legal evidence during the maturation of the retina and the assessment of the response to ocular therapy. In 9% of surviving infants, periventricular hemorrhage occurs.

Outcomes in children with ROP

The major permanent complications in prematurity are neurological deficits, which include cerebral palsy, mental retardation, and visual impairment or blindness.

The health of babies in the NICU does not end with hospital discharge. The medical tasks only stop when a child is able to join society as a healthy infant who is useful and able to fend for him- or herself. Therefore, a child with these characteristics must be discharged if the parents are informed and know what steps are necessary to care for their babies. Providing information about ROP to the parents of children at risk for visual impairment is not only a right of parents, but it is also important for the development of these children. Family-centered care is now the gold standard for health care in special conditions. For this reason, all agents involved in the medical care of this type of child should be prepared to do so appropriately with this focus.

The major vision development occurs in the first year of life and must be evaluated, especially in premature with ROP, who have an increased risk of various ophthalmic and visual dysfunctions and abnormalities. Connolly [41] compared the results of cryotreatment and laser treatment at the age of 10 years. The long-term outcomes and effects of the recently introduced anti-vascular endothelial growth factor (VEGF) drugs are not yet known. In the 1990s, laser therapy was introduced, and in 2002, the visual outcomes of eyes treated with cryotherapy and laser were compared, with better visual outcomes reported with laser.

Children with severe visual deficits are complex patients because many of them have associated pathologies, and although a therapeutic approach should include interdisciplinary action (e.g., developmental pediatrics, neurology, orthopedic surgery, otolaryngology, visually stimulation, psychology, speech therapy), it is important that the ophthalmologist considers part of their role to be to integrate the opinions and advice of all professionals involved in the diagnosis and treatment of the child [42]. Today, laser therapy is the treatment of choice for regression of ROP in the majority of cases. Despite treatment for aggressive posterior ROP (AP-ROP), a substantial proportion of eyes develop retinal detachments, very likely leading to very poor vision, if any [43, 44]. Anti-VEGF treatment can improve the structural and visual outcomes of AP-ROP, but the long-term systemic and ophthalmic effects are still unknown [45].

ROP is a disease with a high risk of visual impairment, so it should be included among diseases of children with special needs. Visual perceptual deficits, including problems with recognition, orientation, depth perception, perception of movement, and simultaneous perception, are becoming common in prematurely born children and can significantly affect their daily lives.

In the evaluation of children with special needs, there are three main indicators to be considered.

1. State of health: morbidity, growth, degree of vision, level of cognitive development, etc.
2. Functional status: social integration, performance in school, ability to perform activities of daily living, level of autonomy

3. Quality of life: the impact the disease has on the individual, considering the patient's perspective.

During evaluations, the infant must be evaluated in the different aspects of development to determine the level of compromise in each patient.

1. Motor: It is necessary to know the normal pattern and any difference in the ages at which children usually sit, stand, crawl, and walk.
2. Language: Related information should be requested at the time of the acquisition of language with the richness of its content. In all cases, there will be the need to apply interconsultation with an otolaryngologist. It is essential to ensure that the auditory pathway works normally because this is the alternative means that is most important for acquiring information about the environment.
3. Visual performance: It is important to question the parents about the visual performance of children in situations of daily life, that is, if the child smiles at familiar faces, can track objects, collides with furniture and toys, is able to find the parent when the parent enters a room or approaches things to see them, recognizes his or her mother when she enters the room, etc. Infants as young as 3 months of age can perceive moving patterns very well, suggesting that the brain areas responsible for motion processing develop rather early. With ERP (evoked retinal potentials), the visual objective response in babies can be measured.

Visual acuity has no direct relationship with the child's visual function. The best way to evaluate this last factor is to observe the child daily. In a child, it is more important to determine the visual performance and visual acuity. Furthermore, it is decisive to determine how the infant can manage to cope with his or her remaining vision.

Visual acuity should not be the only parameter for determining visual functionality, due to

the large capacity of accommodation that children present, allowing them to magnify the retinal image and to improve the performance of their environment relative to their visual deficits.

To assess visual capacity, numerous technical evaluations of the different optical functions exist, including perceptual lenses that are used for visual stimulation, which confirm how the child uses the visual data obtained from the environment.

4. Social integration: This point aims to detect possible trends of disengagement, difficulty interacting with peers, etc.
5. School history: It should be asked whether the child attends a normal or special school, if he or she has an inclusive teacher, if he or she follows the academic content of the courses, and if he or she reads and what types of books are read, especially the print size that he or she is able to see. The physician should exclude learning problems because parents generally tend to interpret any learning difficulties as being the result of vision impairment.

References

1. Terry TL. Extreme prematurity and fibroblastic overgrowth of persistent vascular sheath behind each crystaline lens. Am J Ophthalmol. 1942;25203–4.
2. Campbell K. Intensive oxygen therapy as a possible cause of retrolental fibroplasia. A clinical approach. Med J. Austr. 1951;2:48–50.
3. Solebo AL, Rhi J. Epidemiology, aetiology and management of visual impairment in children. Arch Dis Child. 2014;99:375–9. doi:10.1136/archdischild-2012-303002.
4. Courtright P, Hutchinson AK, Lewallen S. Visual impairment in children in middle- and lower-income countries. Arch Dis Child. 2011;95:1129–34.
5. Epidemiology, aetiology and management of visual impairment in children. Arch. Dis. Child. 2014;99:4375–9.
6. Gogate P, Kalua K, Courtright P. Blindness in childhood in developing countries: time for reassessment? PLoS Med. 2009;6(12):e1000177. doi:10.1371/journal.pmed.1000177.
7. Darlow BA, Hutchinson JL. Simpson JM, Henderson-Smart DJ, Donoghue DA,

Evans NJ. Variation in rates of severe retinopathy of prematurity among neonatal intensive care units in the Australian and New Zealand Neonatal Network. Br J Ophthalmol. 2005;89(12):1592–6. Comment in: Br J Ophthalmol. 2005;89(12):1547.

8. Räisänen S, Gissler M, Saari J, Kramer M, Heinonen S. Contribution of risk factors to extremely, very and moderately preterm births— register-based analysis of 1,390,742 singleton births. PLoS ONE. 2013;8(4):e60660.

9. Gilbert C, Fielder A, Gordillo L, Quinn G, Semiglia R, Visintin P, Zin A. On behalf of the International NO-ROP Group. characteristics of infants with severe retinopathy of prematurity in countries with low, moderate, and high levels of development: implications for screening programs. Pediatrics. 2005;115(5): e518–25. doi:10.1542/peds.2004-1180.

10. Hellstrom A, Engstrom E, Hard AL, Albertsson-Wikland K, Carlsson B, Niklasson A, et al. Postnatal serum insulin-like growth factor I deficiency is associated with retinopathy of prematurity and other complications of premature birth. Pediatrics. 2003;112:1016–20.

11. McColm JR, Geisen P, Hartnett ME. VEGF isoforms and their expression after a single episode of hypoxia or repeated fluctuations between hyperoxia and hypoxia: relevance to clinical ROP. Mol Vis. 2004;10:512–20.

12. Miller JW. Vascular endothelial growth factor and ocular neovascularization. Am J Pathol. 1997; 151:13–23.

13. Chang H, Larson J, Blencowe H, Y Spong C, Paeds. On behalf of the born too soon preterm prevention analysis group preventing preterm births: analysis of trends and potential reductions with interventions in 39 countries with very high human development index. The Lancet 2013;381(9862):223–34.

14. Kinsey VE. Etiology of retrolental fibroplasia and preliminary report of the cooperative study of retrolental fibroplasia. Tr Am Acad Oph Otol. 1955;59:15–24.

15. Askie LM, Henderson-Smart DJ, Irwig L, Simpson JM. Oxygen-saturation targets and outcomes in extremely preterm infants. N Engl J Med. 2003;349:959–67.

16. Askie L. Optimal oxygen saturations in preterm infants a moving target. Curr Opin Pediatr. 2013;25:188–92.

17. Sophie V, Hans D, Lieve M. Oxygen-induced retinopathy in mices amplification by Neonatal IGF-I déficit and attenuation by IGF-I administration. Pediatr Res. 2009;307–9.

18. Vento M, Moro M, Escrig R, et al. Preterm resuscitation with low oxygen causes less oxidative stress, inflammation, and chronic lung disease. Pediatrics. 2009;124(3):e439–49. doi:10.1542/peds. 2009-0434.

19. Carlo WA, Finer NN, Walsh MC, et al. Target ranges of oxygen saturation in extremely preterm infants. N Engl J Med. 2010;362:1959–69.

20. Chow LC, Wright KW, Sola A. CSMC oxygen administration study group. Can changes in clinical practice decrease the incidence of severe retinopathy of prematurity in very low birth weight infants? Pediatrics. 2003;111:339–45.

21. Darlow BA, Marschner S, et al. Randomized controlled trial of oxygen saturation targets in very preterm infants: Two year outcomes on behalf of the benefits of oxygen saturation targeting-New Zealand (BOOST-NZ) collaborative group. J Pediatr. 2014;165:30–5.

22. SUPPORT Study Group of the Eunice Kennedy Shriver NICHD Neonatal Research Network Carlo WA, Finer NN, Walsh MC, et al. Target ranges of oxygen saturation in extremely preterm infants. N Engl J Med. 2010;362:1959–69.

23. Section on Ophthalmology American Academy of Pediatrics; American Academy of Ophthalmology; American Association for Pediatric Ophthalmology and Strabismus. Screening examination of premature infants for retinopathy of prematurity. Pediatrics. 2006;117(2):572–6. Erratum in: Pediatrics. 2006;118 (3):1324.

24. Early Treatment for Retinopathy of Prematurity Cooperative Group. Revised indications for the treatment of retinopathy of prematurity: results of the early treatment for retinopathy of prematurity randomized trial. Arch Ophthalmol. 2003;121 (12):1684–94. Comment in: Arch Ophthalmol. 2003;121(12):1769–71.

25. Retinopathy of prematurity: guidelines for screening and treatment. The report of a Joint Working Party of The Royal College of Ophthalmologists and the British Association of Perinatal Medicine. Early Hum Dev. 1996;46(3):239–58.

26. Karel A, Christine V, Ingele C, Gunnar N, Anne D, Veerle C, Hugo D. Perinatal growth characteristics and associated risk of developing threshold retinopathy of prematurity. J AAPOS. 2003;7:34–7.

27. Aher SM, Ohlsson A. Early versus late erythropoietin for preventing red blood cell transfusion in preterm and/or low birth weight infants. Cochrane Database Syst Rev. 2006;19:3.

28. Kevin K, Jennifer A, Anthony L. Human recombinant erythropoietin and the incidence of retinopathy of prematurity: A multiple regression model. J AAPOS. 2008;12:233–8.

29. Chen M, Citil A, et al. Infection, oxygen, and immaturity: interacting risk factors for retinopathy of prematurity. Neonatology. 2011;99(2):125–32.

30. Pieh C, Agostini H, Buschbeck C, et al. VEGF-A, VEGFR-1, VEGFR-2 and Tie2 levels in plasma of premature infants: relationship to retinopathy of prematurity. Br J Ophthalmol. 2008;92:689–93.

31. Lôfqviwt C, Anderson E, Sigurdsson J, Enstrônm E Hârd AL, Niklasson A, Smith LE Hellstrôm. A 2006 Longitudilan postnatal weight and insulin-like growth factor I measurements in the prediction of retinopathy of prematurity. Arch Ophtalmol 124; 2006:1711–18.

32. Wallace, J. Kylstra, S. Phillips, J. Hall Poor postnatal weight gain: a risk factor for severe retinopathy of prematurity. JAAPOS. 4(6):343–47.

33. Birch DG, Birch EE, Hoffman DR, Uauy RD. Retinal development in very-low-birth-weight infants fed diets differing in omega-3 fatty acids. IOVS. 1992;33:2365–76.

34. Quiram PA, Capone A Jr Current understanding and management of retinopathy of prematurity. Curr Opin Ophthalmol. 2007;18(3):228–34.

35. Kennedy KA, Ipson MA, Birch DG, et al. Light reduction and the electroretinogram of preterm infants. Arch Dis Child Fetal Neonatal Ed. 1997;76:F168–73.

36. STOP-ROP. Supplemental Therapeutic Oxygen for Prethreshold Retinopathy Of Prematurity, a randomized, controlled trial. I: primary outcomes. Pediatrics. Feb 2000;105(2):295–310.

37. Karen Scott, Kim DY, Wang L. Telemedical diagnosis of retinopathy of prematurity. Ophthalmology. 2008;115:1222–8.

38. Lorenz & Katerina Spasovska & Heike Elflein & Nico Schneider. Wide-field digital imaging based telemedicine for screening for acute retinopathy of prematurity (ROP). Six-year results of a multicentre field study. Graefes Arch Clin Exp Ophthalmol. 2009;247:1251–62.

39. Photo-ROP. Cooperative Group Photographic Screening for Retinopathy of Prematurity. The photographic screening for retinopathy of prematurity study (photo-ROP). Primary outcomes. Retina. 2008 Mar;28(3 Suppl):S47–54. Erratum in: Retina. 2009 Jan;29(1):127.

40. Rijken M. Mortality and neurologic, mental, and psychomotor development at 2 years in infants born less than 27 weeks' gestation: the Leiden follow-up project on prematurity. Pediatrics. 2003;112 (2):351–8.

41. Connolly BP, Ng EY, McNamara JA, et al. A comparison of laser photocoagulation with cryotherapy for threshold retinopathy of prematurity at 10 years of age. Ophthalmology. 2002;109:936–41.

42. Ng EY, Connolly BP, McNamara JA, et al. A comparison of laser photocoagulation with cryotherapy for threshold retinopathy of prematurity at 10 years: part 1: visual function and structural outcome. Ophthalmology. 2002;109:928–34.

43. Gunn DJ, Cartwright DW, Yuen SA, et al. Treatment of retinopathy of prematurity in extremely premature infants over an 18 year period. Clin Experiment Ophthalmol. 2013;41(2):159–66.

44. Sanghi G, Dogra MR, Katoch D, et al. Aggressive posterior retinopathy of prematurity: risk factors for retinal detachment despite confluent laser photocoagulation. Am J Ophthalmol. 2013;155(1):159–164.e2.

45. Mintz-Hittner HA, Kennedy KA, Chuang AZ. BEAT-ROP Cooperative Group. Efficacy of intravitreal bevacizumab for stage 31 retinopathy of prematurity. N Engl J Med. 2011;364(7):603–15.

Index

Note: Page numbers with *f* and *t* indicate figures and tables, respectively.

The manufacturer's authorised representative in the EU is Springer
Nature Customer Service Centre GmbH, Europaplatz 3, 69115 Heidelberg,
Germany. If you have any concerns regarding our products, please
contact ProductSafety@springernature.com

Printed and bound by CPI Group (UK) Ltd, Croydon, CR0 4YY
20/04/2026
02093310-0007